AIDS

Science and Society

HUNG FAN

ROSS F. CONNER

LUIS P. VILLARREAL

University of California, Irvine

JONES AND BARTLETT PUBLISHERS

Sudbury, Massachusetts

Boston   London   Singapore

Editorial, Sales, and Customer Service Offices
Jones and Bartlett Publishers
One Exeter Plaza
Boston, MA 02116
617-859-3900
800-832-0034

Jones and Bartlett Publishers International
7 Melrose Terrace
London W6 7RS
England

Portions of this book first appeared in *The Biology of AIDS, Third Edition*, by Hung
Fan, Ross F. Conner, and Luis P. Villarreal © 1994 by Jones and Bartlett Publishers.

Library of Congress Cataloging-in-Publication Data
Fan, Hung, 1947–
    AIDS: science and society/Hung Fan, Ross F. Conner, and Luis
        P. Villarreal.
            p.   cm.
        Includes index.
        ISBN 0-86720-913-5
        1. AIDS (Disease)   I. Conner, Ross F.   II. Villarreal, Luis P.
    III. Title.
    RC607.A26F353   1995   95-9108
    616.97'92—dc20   CIP

Acquisitions Editor: David Phanco
Assistant Production Manager/Coordinator: Judy Songdahl
Manufacturing Buyer: Dana L. Cerrito
Editorial Production Service: Colophon
Cover Design: Hannus Design Associates
Cover Printing: New England Book Components
Printing and Binding: Edwards Brothers, Inc.

Printed in the United States of America

99 98 97 96 95   10 9 8 7 6 5 4 3 2 1

To our HIV-infected friends and acquaintances who are courageously battling the disease or who have succumbed to it. In their honor, and to hasten the day when this book is no longer necessary, a portion of the royalties from this book will be donated to foundations and community organizations dedicated to AIDS research and service.

Contents

CHAPTER 1

Introduction: An Overview of AIDS   1

CHAPTER 2

Concepts of Infectious Disease and a History of Epidemics   7

CHAPTER 3

The Immune System   23

CHAPTER 4

Virology and Human Immunodeficiency Virus   51

CHAPTER 5

Clinical Manifestations of AIDS   79

CHAPTER 6

Epidemiology and AIDS   103

CHAPTER 11

Future Directions in Combating AIDS   213

Preface

The purpose of this text is to provide the nonspecialized student with a firm overview of AIDS from biomedical and psychosocial perspectives. The biological aspects include cellular and molecular descriptions of the immune system and the AIDS virus (Human Immunodeficiency Virus, or HIV). The consequences of HIV infection from cell to organism are also covered, along with a clinical description of the disease. We then move from the organism level to the interorganism level covering both the psychological and social aspects of HIV and AIDS. These topics can only be covered in a survey fashion due to the comprehensive nature of this approach and the additional aim of making this text appropriate for a one-quarter (or semester) course (or part of such a course). We have selected an approach that focuses first on presenting the relevant fundamental principles. Following a brief presentation of these principles for each particular topic, we generalize and apply these concepts to the case of AIDS.

This book incorporates and updates the third edition of *The Biology of AIDS* and also includes consideration of social issues related to HIV and AIDS: personal risk assessment, HIV prevention, and the human and societal dimensions of living with HIV and AIDS. We have provided the latest statistics on AIDS that were available as this book went to press.

This book is patterned after a one-quarter course, AIDS Fundamentals, taught at the University of California, Irvine. Approximately half the course covers biomedical aspects of AIDS, and the other part covers social issues raised by the disease. The text represents the material covered in the course. At

UCI, AIDS Fundamentals is open to all undergraduate students and is taught assuming that they have had a high school level modern-biology course. The material covered in Chapters 3 (immunology), 4 (virology), 6 (epidemiology), 9 (preventing HIV), and 10 (living with HIV and AIDS) is covered in three hours of lecture per chapter. Material covered in the other chapters is taught in a single one-and-a-half hour lecture per chapter. We have found that the students are able to assimilate and retain the material when delivered at this rate. The course includes another important component: small discussion groups led by students who previously took the class. These peer-led groups use experiential exercises as a catalyst for a deeper understanding of the human and social aspects of HIV and AIDS.

Most researchers and scholars in AIDS-related fields were unprepared for the dramatic impact of the emerging AIDS epidemic. As virologists and social scientists, we might have expected modern biomedical technology to provide a quick technical solution or to at least prevent, via vaccine development, the spread of this major new viral epidemic. It is now clear that even though this technology has hastened biomedical progress in AIDS, the AIDS epidemic poses new and unforeseen difficulties with no quick biological solution in sight. These difficulties challenge both our scientific abilities and the ability of our society to respond appropriately. It is our goal to provide students with a conceptual framework of the issues raised by the AIDS epidemic so that they will be better able to deal with the challenges posed by this disease. This is particularly important because new information about scientific aspects of AIDS appears almost daily; with this information come new implications for the clinical, social, psychological, legal, and ethical aspects of the disease. We hope that the framework provided in this book will help students understand and make informed decisions about AIDS-related issues as they develop in the future.

Acknowledgments

We wish to thank David Fan, Elaine Vaughan, Michael Gorman, David Prescott, Cedric Davern, David Baltimore, and Frank Lilly for reading parts of the manuscript prior to publication and providing many helpful substantive and editorial comments. Juan Moreno applied outstanding computer graphic skills in generating all the line drawings for the book, Arthur Durazo assisted with Spanish translation, and Mirella Marinelli provided speedy and accurate word-processing assistance. Bob Settineri of Sierra Productions was of great help in obtaining the other figures. Paula Carroll, Helen Shaw of Colophon, Deborah Haffner, and other editorial staff of Jones and Bartlett were responsible for production of the final volume. We are grateful for their assistance and gentle prodding. We also wish to thank Michael Feldman and Emmett Carlson for their love and support.

Authors

Dr. Hung Fan is Professor of Virology in the Department of Molecular Biology and Biochemistry at the University of California, Irvine and Director of the UCI Cancer Research Institute. His research interest is in how retroviruses cause disease and induce cancer and AIDS.

Dr. Ross Conner is Associate Professor, Department of Urban and Regional Planning, School of Social Ecology, and Department of Medicine, School of Medicine at the University of California, Irvine. Dr. Conner's research interest is in the evaluation of the effectiveness of public and social programs, particularly health promotion programs, including HIV prevention.

Dr. Luis Villarreal is Professor of Virology in the Department of Molecular Biology and Biochemistry at the University of California, Irvine. Dr. Villarreal's research interest is in the strategy of how viruses replicate and how they cause disease.

Chapter 1

Introduction:
An Overview of AIDS

AIDS IN BRIEF

THE AIDS EPIDEMIC

A report appeared in 1981 that initially drew little attention from infectious disease experts. In that report, Dr. Michael Gottlieb, at the University of California at Los Angeles, described a rare form of pneumonia occurring in homosexual men. Other reports from about the same time indicated that other homosexual men were developing rare forms of cancer. This new set of symptoms, a *syndrome* in medical terms, was eventually called *Acquired Immune Deficiency Syndrome* because the symptoms were consistent with damage to the immune system in previously healthy individuals. Moreover, this disease was not congenital or inherited but appeared to have been acquired. We now know that this resulted from infection by a virus. Since then, the acronym *AIDS*, which is used to describe this disease, has become a prominent and permanent fixture in our language. It evokes a range of responses, including fear, hate, and mistrust. Some of these responses (hate, mistrust) are related to the association of AIDS with subcultural groups within our society, such as male homosexuals, who already have experienced discrimination. Other responses (fear) are due to the grave nature of the AIDS disease and the threat it may pose to society. This is because the AIDS epidemic continues to grow—unlike most other major infectious diseases that have been controlled by a combination of clinical treatments and public health measures.

AIDS IN BRIEF

We now know that AIDS is caused by *Human Immunodeficiency Virus (HIV)*, but it was originally observed by its effects on the immune system. An important clue was that AIDS patients often developed a lung infection (or pneumonia) caused by fungus called *Pneumocystis carinii*. This infection is very rare in healthy individuals, but patients with cancers of the immune system itself (lymphomas) were known to be susceptible to this disease. Lymphomas are usually treated by chemotherapy, which is intended to destroy the cancer cells. However, chemotherapy also will unavoidably destroy many healthy immune cells along with the cancerous lymphoma cells. Thus, this type of pneumonia predominantly occurs in patients with a damaged immune system. Examination of AIDS patients confirmed that their immune systems were damaged. The specific nature of this damage is discussed in greater detail in Chapters 3 and 4. It had been known for some time that various other viral infections could damage cells of the immune system, but such severe damage as is seen with AIDS was unprecedented. Although doctors suspected early on that AIDS resulted from infection by a virus, it was not until 1984 that the virus was finally isolated by both French and American researchers. That virus is now known as *HIV*.

In addition to pneumonia, AIDS is associated with numerous other infections. These secondary infections are caused by various bacteria, protozoa, fungi, and other viruses. Usually, it is these infections (known as *opportunistic infections*) that cause death in AIDS patients. In addition to secondary infections, AIDS patients frequently develop cancers, including *lymphomas* and an otherwise rare cancer called *Kaposi's sarcoma*. HIV infection also can result in damage to brain cells. This leads to loss of mental function, referred to as *AIDS dementia*. A more complete description of the clinical features of AIDS is presented in Chapter 5. Most of these opportunistic infections and some other effects of HIV infection can be explained by damage to the immune system.

HIV causes disease insidiously. The early stages of infection are often not apparent, without any visible symptoms. The infected person may feel healthy and appears to be completely normal during this time (the incubation period) but such a person is able to transmit the infection. The HIV incubation period is of variable duration and can be quite long (on average 8 to 10 years). In contrast, for most common virus infections, such as colds or influenza, an incubation period of a few days or weeks will be followed by apparent disease. This adds greatly to the difficulty of studying and controlling AIDS, because many people infected with the virus have not yet developed the disease.

THE AIDS EPIDEMIC

Despite the many different clinical symptoms that result from AIDS, medical investigators have already learned a great deal about how AIDS is spread in our population. For example, it is now clear that HIV transmission requires close contact and that infection occurs by one of three routes: blood, birth, or sex. Casual contact does not lead to disease transmission. AIDS epidemiology is further discussed in Chapter 6.

Between 1981 (the beginning of the AIDS epidemic) and the end of 1992, about 240,000 cases of AIDS in the United States were reported to the National Centers for Disease Control (CDC) in Atlanta, Georgia. Of these cases, about 160,000 (67 percent) have died. Sexually active homosexual males were originally the major afflicted group and represent about 60 percent of these reported cases. Another 21 percent of the cases were male or female intravenous drug users, and 7 percent were male homosexual drug users. The remaining 12 percent resulted from heterosexual transmission, birth, or by blood transfusion during the period when the American blood supply was not monitored for HIV antibodies (1981–1985).

The AIDS epidemic is not restricted to the United States. It can be found on all continents and hence is considered a *pandemic.* There may be as many as 10 million people in sub-Saharan Africa who are infected with HIV. In Africa, HIV transmission predominantly results from heterosexual contact and other modes. Given the relatively poor medical support available in much of Africa, the number of infected people may increase significantly. Very recently, HIV infection has been spreading explosively in South Asia as well, with Thailand and India strongly affected. As there is no cure for AIDS, these numbers are alarming. They indicate the clear potential of AIDS to spread unchecked, in spite of recent advances in modern medicine, epidemiology, virology, and recombinant DNA technology. This reminds us of previous times when major infectious diseases devastated human populations (see Chapter 2). How can we control this epidemic? An overview of the relationship between epidemics and human populations may shed some light on this.

Chapter 2

Concepts of Infectious Disease and a History of Epidemics

FACTORS THAT AFFECT THE SPREAD OF EPIDEMICS

- Host and Virus Populations
- The Transmission Rate
- Population Densities and Infections
- Chronic Infections
- Controlling Infectious Diseases

A HISTORY OF EPIDEMICS

- The Old World
- The New World
- Modern Concepts of Infectious Disease
- Epidemics in Modern Times
- Syphilis: The Social Problems with a Sexually Transmitted Disease

One of the great recent achievements of modern civilization has been the control of infectious diseases. It is likely that few of us, for example, personally know someone who died from a contagious disease. In historical terms, however, this is a new development, one that occurred in this century. In previous centuries, death from infectious disease was common, and whole populations were often affected.

When a population becomes infected with a contagious disease, an epidemic results. *Epidemic* is derived from Greek and means "in one place among the people." To understand how an infectious disease can spread or remain established in a population, we must consider the relationship between an infectious disease agent and its host population. The study of diseases in populations is an area of medicine known as *epidemiology,* which will be further discussed in Chapter 6.

We now know that contagious diseases are spread by microorganisms, such as certain bacteria and viruses, which cause disease when they infect a susceptible person. This is a modern concept, known as the *germ theory* of infectious disease. As we shall see, earlier societies often used moral or religious explanations for infectious disease, and their social behavior reflected those beliefs.

FACTORS THAT AFFECT THE SPREAD OF EPIDEMICS

In this section, we shall discuss factors that influence the spread of infectious diseases. While various microorganisms cause disease, and the general principles are the same, we will concentrate on viruses, since HIV is a virus.

Host and Virus Populations

An epidemic consists of infection of a number of individuals in a population. It is important to look at more than a single person in order to understand how diseases spread. Two populations must be considered: the human host and the infecting agent—in the case of AIDS, a virus. These two populations have a balanced parasite-host relationship. A viral infection can deplete or limit the population of its host, but a highly lethal virus that spreads rapidly might kill all available hosts and lead to the extinction of both its host and itself. The outcome of an epidemic, however, is not always straightforward and can vary according to a number of other factors that relate to the population. These factors include:

1. the total number of hosts
2. their birth rate
3. the rate at which susceptible individuals migrate into the population
4. the number of susceptible hosts who are not infected
5. the rate at which the disease can be transmitted from an infected individual to an uninfected one
6. the number of infected individuals who die
7. the number who survive the infection and become immune or resistant to further infection.

Figure 2–1 shows a schematic relationship between infected and uninfected people for a simple acute infection; all infected individuals either recover from the disease and become immune to it or they die from it. The arrows that connect the boxed groups represent movement of people from one group to

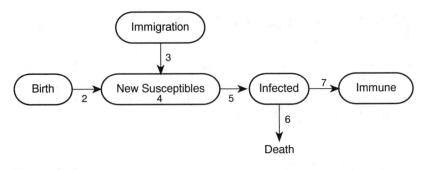

Figure 2–1

Population factors that affect epidemics: 1. Population size; 2. Birth rate; 3. Immigration rate; 4. Number of susceptibles; 5. Transmission rate; 6. Death rate; 7. Immune rate.

an adjacent one. This scheme is a simplified representation of the dynamics or ecology of a virus epidemic. It is possible to develop mathematical models to describe or predict an epidemic if the rates of movement through the scheme can be determined. One of the applications of the field of epidemiology (see Chapter 6) is to determine these rates.

The Transmission Rate

The arrow in Figure 2–1 that connects the susceptibles to the infected group is the *transmission rate* of infection. This *rate* represents the efficiency with which disease is transmitted from an infected to a susceptible person. This transmission rate has two major components (Figure 2–2). One is the *inherent efficiency* with which a specific virus can infect a susceptible person. The inherent efficiency of a virus is dependent on the biological properties of the virus as well as the route by which the virus enters the susceptible person. For example, influenza virus, like many other respiratory viruses, has a high inherent efficiency of infection and is highly contagious. Respiratory viruses are easily taken up by breathing in aerosols (sneezes), and once influenza virus comes into contact with cells of the respiratory tract, it readily infects them. HIV, on the other hand, actually has a relatively poor inherent infection efficiency, as we shall see later.

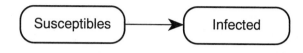

Figure 2-2

Transmission rate of infections: 1. Inherent efficiency of virus infection; 2. Encounter rate between infected and uninfected.

The other major component of the transmission rate is the rate at which a susceptible person encounters an infectious person—the *encounter rate*. Each encounter between an infected and an uninfected person increases the likelihood that an infection will be transmitted.

As we shall see later with the AIDS virus, both of these components of transmission can be changed by altering the behavior of susceptible and infected persons. Behaviors that allow high encounter rates with infected people or that allow more efficient infection will favor the spread of an epidemic. Conversely, changes in behavior that reduce these transmission factors may control the spread of an epidemic.

Population Densities and Infections

Many of the epidemics that have plagued mankind for the last few thousand years would not have had a favorable transmission rate during early human civilization. Early human societies were not urban but consisted of hunter-gatherers who lived in relatively small groups, such as extended families. Such small groups or small populations cannot produce new susceptibles in high enough numbers at any given time to support the continued presence of many epidemic disease microorganisms. An acute disease will produce symptoms and make a person infectious soon after infection. The infected person will transmit the disease, die from the infection, or recover and become immune to subsequent infections. An acute microorganism that strikes such small groups will quickly infect all available susceptibles and then die out.

About 10,000 years ago, the agricultural revolution allowed human populations to become large enough to support epidemics. In other words, the development of human civilization was necessary before epidemics by acute viruses could establish stable footholds. When the world population became sufficiently large, different patterns of infection also could develop. Epidemic diseases could establish an *endemic* pattern—one in which the disease is always present. Following the initial introduction and spread into a susceptible or naïve population, even a very lethal virus can become endemic. In an endemic disease, the numbers who are actively infected are much lower, but the virus is always present in the population. Endemic viral diseases are often considered childhood diseases because the virus is so common in the population that most individuals encounter it during childhood. Most adults have had the disease and survived. This may be related to the high infant mortality of previous eras (Europe in the Dark and Middle Ages) and to high infant mortality in some developing countries today. Endemic infectious agents can limit population sizes and result in populations that are relatively unaffected or resistant to the infectious agent as a whole. As we shall see below, this can have major consequences when two previously separated societies encounter each other for the first time.

Chronic Infections

In addition to acute infections, such as measles, there are also chronic infections. In *acute infections*, the disease symptoms generally occur quite soon after infection, and the infectious agent is generally eliminated from the individual after the initial disease period. However, even some people infected with an acute virus will not develop symptoms (subclinical infections). In a *chronic infection*, the person does not eradicate the infectious agent (often a virus). The virus persists in the infected person and may be produced at low levels. People with chronic infections often will not show symptoms or disease immediately after infection. The differences between acute infection and chronic infection in an infected individual are diagrammed in Figure 2–3. As described above, acute infections generally require large populations (with continued new susceptibles) in order to be maintained. In contrast, chronic infections can sometimes be maintained in small

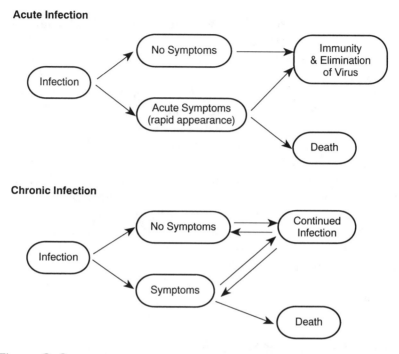

Figure 2–3

Acute vs. chronic infection. The consequences of infection of an individual by an acute virus, compared to infection by a chronic virus. The frequencies with which death, immunity, or continued infection occur are different for different viruses.

populations. In addition, chronic infections are often more difficult to control because infected and uninfected people may be indistinguishable. As we shall see below, the syphilis epidemic was difficult to control partly because it is a chronic infection. Like syphilis, AIDS also results from chronic infection.

Controlling Infectious Diseases

Since the turn of this century, there has been a steady and dramatic decrease in the number of people who die from infectious diseases. Recently, most developed countries have been free of major lethal contagious diseases. Antibiotics can kill bacterial infections after they start. Viruses pose a different problem: They are difficult to eliminate once they become established. Therefore, viral diseases have been controlled mostly by vaccination (see Chapter 4) but occasionally by other measures. A vaccine interrupts the flow of new susceptibles from newborns into the susceptible subpopulation by making young people immune to a virus before they become infected by it (Figure 2–4). If enough (but not necessarily all) susceptibles become immunized, this confers immunity to the population as a whole. This is because the remaining unimmunized but susceptible individuals are unlikely to encounter another infectious individual. It is possible to eliminate some diseases completely from the human population with an effective vaccination program. The smallpox virus, which was responsible for so much human death in historic times, is now eradicated due to successful worldwide vaccination efforts.

A HISTORY OF EPIDEMICS

The Old World

Even the very earliest historical records document the major impact of epidemics. It is not always clear to us now which infectious agent was causing a particular epidemic in ancient times, but we

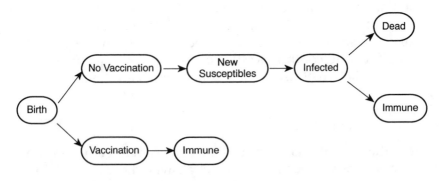

Figure 2–4

Epidemic control by vaccination.

can often make guesses from the recorded symptoms. The three disease agents that have probably caused most human deaths are smallpox virus, measles virus, and the plague bacterium, *Yersinia pestis*. These three diseases have accounted for hundreds of millions of human deaths over the years and an unfathomable amount of human suffering. Other important epidemic agents include influenza virus, typhoid fever bacterium, yellow fever virus, polio virus, and, more recently, hepatitis virus. The syphilis bacterium *Treponema pallidum* is of special interest here due to its sexual mode of transmission and its associated social problems.

Many historical accounts make clear reference to a supposed religious or moral reason for a particular epidemic. The transmission of disease itself was often believed to occur through casting of an evil eye. In the Old Testament, for example, Moses brought onto the Egyptians a plague of "sores that break into pustules" due to the sins of the Egyptians. Epidemics were often perceived as punishment due to the wrath of a deity, perhaps for some offense by the entire population. Those who developed a disease were viewed as deserving it. This tendency to link a disease to social stigmatism has persisted throughout history and afflicts people with AIDS today.

The Greek writings are probably the earliest accounts in sufficient detail to allow us to measure the impact of epidemic disease. Aside from malaria, the Greeks were relatively free of most infectious diseases with one important exception. In 430–429 B.C., an epidemic that may have been measles struck Athens with a devastating loss of life. It also resulted in a significant decrease in the size of its armies—and the following year Athens lost a war with Sparta. Thus, this epidemic may have influenced history.

The Roman Empire also suffered massive epidemics in 165 A.D. and again in 251 A.D. Prior to the 165 A.D. epidemic, population of the Roman Empire was probably at its peak (about 54 million). After the 165 A.D. and 251 A.D. epidemics, the Roman population did not recover its size until modern times. The first epidemic could have been smallpox and appears to have killed one third of Rome's population. The 251 A.D. epidemic may have been due to measles and was equally devastating: There were about 5,000 deaths per day in Rome at its peak. Rome's rural population may have been even more affected. This die-off may have led to the depopulation of agricultural lands and an inability to oppose invasion from the north. A third massive epidemic occurred in 542–543 A.D., probably due to bubonic plague. Soon after this plague, Rome's armies fell to the Visigoth and then the Moslem armies, and the Dark Age of Europe began. Thus, epidemiological history suggests that infectious diseases may have contributed to the fall of the Roman Empire.

The situation for the Han Chinese society, although more difficult to estimate, appears to have been similar. Massive epidemics in 162 A.D. and again in 310 A.D. may account for much of the population decline in China, which peaked at about 50 million at those times but declined to about 8.9 million by 742 A.D.

In Europe, and probably also in China, measles and smallpox eventually became endemic childhood diseases following these devastating epidemics. In the following millennia, Europe experienced devastating epidemics from the disease known as the *black death*. Black death was a pneumonic form (or lung infection) of plague, which had a very high fatality rate. It probably accounted for up to 100 million deaths in Europe. The worst of these epidemics occurred in 1346. This epidemic appears to have been a *pandemic*, meaning that other continents (China and India) were also involved. The black death recurred in Europe in the 1360s and again in the 1370s. The seemingly arbitrary pattern of death and the massive suffering had dark social consequences for Europe. Xenophobia, the fear of foreigners, became common. Violent riots against Jews and Gypsies occurred in numerous cities, as they were blamed as a source of the plague. Self-flagellation became a common practice and rational theology lost popular acceptance. The situation improved somewhat in the 1400s. Black death became endemic, possibly because of selection for a less virulent plague bacterium; selection for people with greater resistance to the disease also may have occurred. European society was now experiencing most of these acute infectious diseases, especially the viral diseases, as childhood diseases.

The New World

A well-documented example of what happens when a new viral disease enters a naïve population (one that has never encountered the virus) occurred when Cortez went to Mexico and introduced smallpox into the New World. The Aztec Codices (hieroglyphic-like records) tell us that the New World was relatively free of major infectious disease at that time. The population of Mexico was probably 25–30 million, and Mexico City may then have been the most populous city in the world. In 1518, just as the Aztecs drove off Cortez from Mexico City, a smallpox epidemic swept though the city, killing the Aztec leaders and decimating the city's population. This epidemic was followed by numerous other diseases that were endemic European childhood diseases but were devastating to the Aztecs. Within 50 years, the population of Mexico was down to about 1.5 million, or about 5 percent of what it had been at its peak. Furthermore, the fact that the diseases seemed to strike only the Aztecs and not the Spaniards led the Aztecs to believe that the gods favored the Spaniards.

Other American natives fared even worse than the Aztecs: The Indians of Baja, California and other island tribes became totally extinct. Thus, the main fabric of native American society was utterly destroyed. Mexico only began to recover from this population loss in the 1800s, and only now has Mexico City become the most populous city in the world again. A similar fate was in store for the Pacific island natives, who also suffered huge population losses after encountering European explorers. Thus, throughout human history, infectious diseases have profoundly affected human populations.

Modern Concepts of Infectious Disease

The germ theory of infection was first proposed in 1546 by Girolamo Fracatoro, a Franciscan monk. However, it was not until the 1840s that H. Henle, a German physician, clarified these concepts and they became accepted among scientists. One of Henle's students, Robert Koch, subsequently proposed four postulates that could be used to prove that an infectious agent causes a disease. This was a milestone in the understanding of infectious disease. Koch's postulates state that an organism can be considered to cause a disease if it fulfills the following criteria:

1. The organism is always found in diseased individuals.
2. The organism can be isolated from the diseased individual and grown pure in culture.

3. The pure culture will initiate and reproduce the disease when introduced back into a susceptible host (either man or animal).
4. The organism can be reisolated from the diseased individual.

These postulates allowed scientifically sound assignments of what agents caused specific diseases, and they freed physicians from many superstitions and myths that had historically prevailed.

Actually, by today's standards, Koch's postulates are sometimes too stringent. For example, viruses cannot be grown pure in culture in the absence of cells (see Chapter 4). Also, if two infectious agents cooperate to cause a disease or a particular set of symptoms, it would also be impossible to fulfill Koch's postulates. We shall see that this situation applies to HIV infection and AIDS. In the late 1800s, however, such stringency was necessary.

The timing of the development of Koch's postulates, and of the development of the science of epidemiology, was most fortunate because other changes in society set the stage for the outbreak of another worldwide epidemic. In the late 1800s, steamships brought about relatively rapid world travel. This change had an impact on the ecology of infectious disease by allowing the rapid movement of infected persons who could quickly spread an epidemic. In 1894, another plague pandemic broke out, initially in Burma, then in Hong Kong, then via steamships to all major ports worldwide, including those in the United States. By applying the germ theory of disease and epidemiology, society was able to respond to this threat. The application of Koch's postulates led to the rapid identification and isolation of the causative bacterium, *Yersinia pestis*. Furthermore, intense epidemiological studies identified rats, and more specifically their fleas, as major carriers of the disease. This led to the development of preventative measures to control the spread of the plague, principally by limiting interactions between rats and humans. Except for a further breakout in India, the plague epidemic was stopped. This was an important lesson. There was no cure or vaccine for plague at this time, yet understanding the routes of infection and designing measures based on this understanding to minimize spread of infection averted a pandemic. With the current AIDS epidemic we are in a similar situation, because there is no cure or vaccine. Behavior modification to minimize spread of AIDS virus is currently our only means of controlling the epidemic. However, because AIDS is predominantly a sexually transmitted disease, modification of behavior is difficult.

Epidemics in Modern Times

In the twentieth century, several other epidemics have taken a toll on humanity. During the great pandemic of 1918, influenza virus killed about 20 million people worldwide and virtually brought World War I to a halt. About 80 percent of American casualties in World War I were due to influenza, a fact seldom mentioned in most history texts. Influenza continues to cause epidemics and remains a health threat. The major reason is because this virus can mutate rapidly. These mutations lead to changes in the surface structure of the virus that allow the virus to avoid the protection of the immune system. As a result, individuals who were previously infected with influenza virus are not protected from the new mutant virus. As we will see later, HIV also has a similar property.

Poliovirus is another recent epidemic disease. This disease appeared as a new viral epidemic in the United States in 1894—much as the AIDS epidemic appeared in 1981. Poliovirus can damage the nervous system and lead to paralysis. In contrast to HIV, which entered North America in the late 1970s (see Chapter 4), poliovirus had been infecting people since early history, but it did not cause documented epidemics until 1894. We now believe that improvements in hygiene and sanitation occurring in more developed societies actually predisposed individuals to the paralytic form of polio by delaying exposure to the virus until they were young adults. Infection of infants, which tends to occur in less developed countries, usually results in a mild nonparalytic gastrointestinal infection. Thus, the people most likely to get paralytic polio were the healthy young adults from the highest socioeconomic classes. This demonstrates the unforeseen effects that changes in social behavior can have on the ecology of an epidemic. Polio had a major impact on the American consciousness, as seen by highly visible national crusades during the first half of the twentieth century (such as the March of Dimes). This underlines the way that the nature of the victims can influence public perceptions of a disease and society's response to it. In fact, there were about 50,000 total deaths from paralytic polio during the first half of this century. It is interesting to contrast the public response to polio during this time to recent responses to AIDS—even though more deaths from AIDS have occurred in the first ten years of the epidemic.

Syphilis: The Social Problems with a Sexually Transmitted Disease

One epidemic that is hauntingly similar to the AIDS epidemic is syphilis. The parallels are striking. At the time of the syphilis epidemic, scientific investigation of this insidious disease was at the leading edge of medicine and microbiology, as is the current situation with AIDS. The issues raised included public health policy and civil liberties, again as in the AIDS epidemic. And finally, because it is a sexually transmitted disease, syphilis patients were highly stigmatized. A cure for syphilis in infected individuals was developed in 1909, but it was not until the 1940s that the epidemic was finally controlled.

Why did it take so long to control this epidemic? Like AIDS, syphilis can be a long-term and variable disease, with phases in which no symptoms are apparent. Unfortunately, untreated syphilis often eventually leads to death. More important, at the time syphilis was perceived as a social problem—hence the reference to it as a *social disease.* Many blamed the disease on a breakdown of social values and promoted the view that a sexual ethic in which all sex was marital and monogamous would make it impossible to acquire the disease. The initial public health policies to control this epidemic were based on these views. Abstinence from extramarital sexual contact was encouraged, and prostitution was repressed since prostitutes were blamed as the major source of infection of otherwise monogamous males. Immigrants were also blamed for bringing the disease from abroad, even though epidemiological data did not support this view. As many as 20,000 prostitutes were quarantined or jailed during World War I. In addition, the Army discouraged the availability of condoms for fear that they might encourage soldiers to engage in extramarital sex. There were also campaigns to stigmatize soldiers who became infected with syphilis by giving them dishonorable discharges. These policies were not based on epidemiological evidence, and they failed to control the epidemic, which actually grew during this period.

It was not until the 1930s that the surgeon general of the United States, Thomas Parren, proposed major changes in the public health approaches to control the syphilis epidemic. These policy changes were ultimately successful but required substantial funding from Congress. The proposals called for the elimination of repressive approaches that discouraged people from participating in programs or seeking treatment. Free and confidential diagnostic and treatment centers were set up throughout the nation. A national educational campaign was begun to educate the public and dispel prevalent misconceptions (even among respected sources) about its transmission. Syphilis is transmitted by sexual contact but not by casual contact. These policies, along with new antibiotics, brought the syphilis epidemic under control in the 1940s.

With the AIDS epidemic, we are dealing with powerful biological drives such as human sexuality and drug addiction. The syphilis epidemic shows us that policies based mainly on abstinence are not very effective in controlling a sexually transmitted disease. Other alterations in behavior will be necessary to reduce the transmission of AIDS and bring this epidemic under control. Until a cure or a vaccine against AIDS is developed, changing behavior (see Chapter 9) is our most effective means of controlling the AIDS pandemic.

Chapter 3

The Immune System

BLOOD

- Cells of the Blood

THE LYMPHATIC CIRCULATION

B-CELLS AND HUMORAL IMMUNITY

- How Does the Immune System Respond to New Antigens?
- The Primary Immune Response
- A Secondary Immune Response
- A Summary of the Humoral Immune System

T-CELLS AND CELL-MEDIATED IMMUNITY

- T_{killer} Lymphocytes
- T_{helper} Lymphocytes

As mentioned in Chapter 1, AIDS results from a viral infection that ultimately disables the immune system. In order to understand this disease, we need to understand the immune system. This system is an intricate collection of cells and fluids in our body that gives us the ability to fight off infections. HIV, the AIDS virus, specifically affects certain cells of the immune system. Once we know about these cells and what they do, we can see how HIV does its damage. This chapter provides a simplified overview of immunity—many more intricacies and details are known, but the information provided here will allow us to understand the basic immunological problems associated with AIDS.

BLOOD

In order to understand the immune system, we must first consider blood. Blood is a system of circulating cells and fluids that carries out many important functions for the body. These functions include *transport of nutrients and oxygen* to the body tissues, *elimination of waste products and carbon dioxide* from tissues, *wound repair,* and *protection from infection by foreign agents.* Besides cells, the fluid portion of blood contains many different substances and molecules that help carry out these functions. Some examples are sugars that are necessary for energy metabolism in our tissues, and antibodies, which are important in fighting infections. The cell-free fluid portion of blood is referred to as *plasma.* Serum can be obtained from isolated blood by letting it stand and clot; the cells are trapped in the clot and can be removed easily.

Cells and substances of the blood that are responsible for protection from infection make up the *immune system*. The immune system must protect us from a wide variety of infectious agents. These include (in ascending order of complexity):

Viruses. These are very small subcellular agents (see Chapter 4).

Bacteria. These are small, single-cell microorganisms, which have relatively simple genetic material. Typhoid fever and tuberculosis are caused by bacteria.

Protozoa. These are single-cell microorganisms that contain more complicated genetic structures. Amoebas and Giardia are examples of protozoa.

Fungi. These are more complex microorganisms that may exist as single cells, or they maybe organized into simple multicellular organisms. Examples are yeasts and molds.

Multicellular Parasites. These can be relatively large organisms, such as roundworms and tapeworms.

In addition, the immune system is also important in fighting cancer.

Blood is carried throughout the body by a series of blood vessels that make up the *circulatory system* (Figure 3–1). The heart is the pump for the circulatory system, and it moves blood through the blood vessels by its rhythmic muscular contractions. There are three kinds of blood vessels: *arteries*, which carry blood away from the heart to the body tissues; *veins*, which carry blood back to the heart from the tissues; and *capillaries*. Capillaries are very thin-walled blood vessels in the tissues that connect the arteries with the veins, and they allow exchange of oxygen, nutrients, and wastes between the blood and tissues. Some kinds of blood cells (such as the white blood cells called *monocytes* and *lymphocytes*) can also pass through these thin walls from the blood into the tissues as well. The lungs are another important part of the circulatory system—this is where the exchange of oxygen and carbon dioxide between the blood and the air we breathe takes place.

The cells in the blood have limited life spans—ranging from one or two days to several weeks, depending on the cell type. This means that they must be continually replenished.

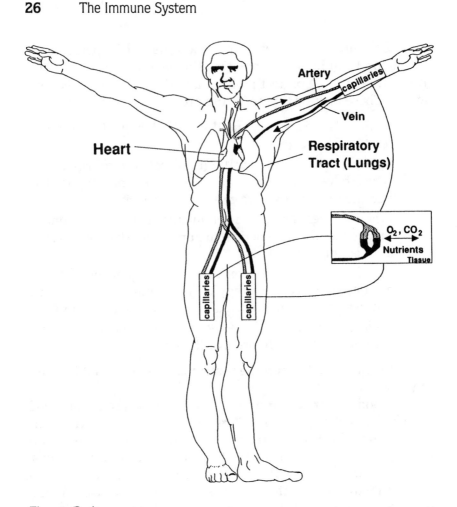

Figure 3–1

The circulatory system.

They are replenished from *stem cells* that are located in the bone marrow. These stem cells have the capacity to divide and make more of themselves, and to differentiate and mature into blood cells of all types (Figure 3–2). During the differentiation process, the stem cells first develop into *committed precursors,* which can either divide or differentiate into mature blood cells of a particular kind. This process goes on throughout life and, if interrupted, results in very serious health problems.

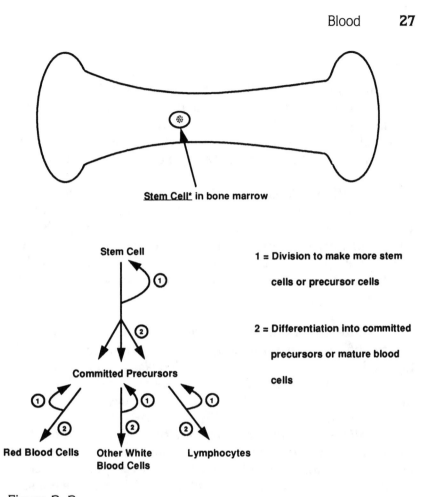

Figure 3–2

Growth and maturation of blood cells.

When stem cells and committed precursors divide or differentiate, they require the presence of *growth factors* in order to carry out these processes. Different growth factors stimulate particular kinds of blood cells, and these growth factors play important roles in regulating the orderly growth and replenishment of all blood cells. For example, interleukin 2 is a growth factor that is required by blood cells called T-lymphocytes, which are discussed later.

Cells of the Blood

Let us now look at the different kinds of cells present in blood. These cells are shown in Figure 3–3. Blood cells are divided into *red blood cells* and *white blood cells*. There are a lot of red blood cells, but they are a single cell type; the white blood cells are fewer in number, but they are made up of many cell types.

Red Blood Cells   Red blood cells or *erythrocytes* are responsible for carrying oxygen to the tissues and carbon dioxide away from them. They contain a protein called *hemoglobin* that binds and carries the oxygen and carbon dioxide within them. Hemoglobin gives red blood cells their characteristic red color. All the other blood cells are called white blood cells, since they lack hemoglobin.

White Blood Cells   White blood cells or *leukocytes* are of several different types. *Megakaryocytes* are very large blood cells that bud off subcellular fragments called *platelets*. Platelets circulate through the bloodstream, and if they encounter a break in a blood vessel they cause a clot to form. Thus, they are involved in wound repair.

Cells of the immune system are of two classes: those that respond to a specific foreign agent or substance and those that are *not* specific for the agent they attack. The cells that are specific for a certain foreign agent are *lymphocytes*. Cells that are not specific for the foreign agent they attack include *phagocytes, mast cells, eosinophils* and *natural killer cells.*

Phagocytes are cells that attack and eliminate foreign cells or bacteria by engulfing or eating them. *Phagein* is the Greek word for "to eat." There are two different kinds of phagocytes: *macrophages* (and related monocytes) and *neutrophils* (also called *phagocytic granulocytes*). Macrophages generally attack and engulf cells infected with viruses, while neutrophils generally attack foreign bacteria. Macrophages are not only found in the blood (where the immature forms are called monocytes), but they also are present in tissues.

Mast cells, basophils, and eosinophils attack infectious agents that are too large to be engulfed by a single blood cell. Such agents include protozoa and large parasites such as worms. Mast

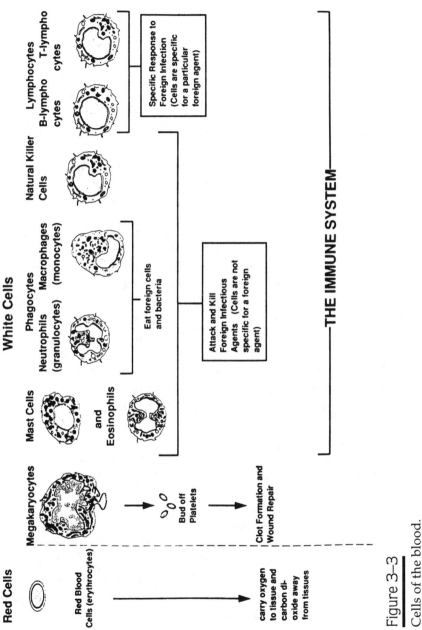

Figure 3-3

Cells of the blood.

cells and eosinophils come into contact with the foreign agents and release toxic compounds that may kill those foreign agents.

What instructs phagocytes, mast cells and eosinophils to attack a foreign agent? In general, *antibodies*, which are proteins produced by certain lymphocytes (see below), first bind to the foreign agent in a specific fashion. The phagocytes, mast cells, or eosinophils then recognize the agent because of the antibodies bound to it, and they attack. This process is diagramed in Figure 3–4.

Lymphocytes are cells that respond *specifically* to particular foreign substances or *antigens*. It is important to define an antigen. An *antigen* is a molecule or substance against which lymphocytes will raise a response. An example of an antigen would be a protein of a virus particle; the number of possible antigens that we might encounter is virtually limitless.

Lymphocytes are divided into two types: B-lymphocytes and T-lymphocytes. *B-lymphocytes* secrete soluble proteins called *antibodies* into the circulatory system. Each individual antibody specifically recognizes and binds to one particular antigen. Once this happens, the antibody signals other cells in the immune system to attack (Figure 3–4). In addition, certain antibodies may bind directly and inhibit the function of infectious agents such as viruses. These are called *neutralizing antibodies.*

T-lymphocytes (or T-cells) make proteins called *receptors* that are similar to antibodies in that these proteins recognize specific antigens. However, T-lymphocytes do not release their receptors but hold them on their cell surfaces. As a result, the T-lymphocytes themselves specifically recognize and bind to foreign antigens.

There are two major kinds of T-lymphocytes: *cytotoxic or killer* T-cells (T_{killer}), and *helper* T-cells (T_{helper}). T_{killer} cells directly bind to cells carrying a foreign antigen. Once they bind to them, they attack and kill those cells, thus eliminating them from the body. T_{helper} cells, on the other hand, do not kill cells. Instead, they interact with B-lymphocytes or T_{killer} lymphocytes and help them respond to antigens (more about this later). In addition to the receptors, T_{killer} and T_{helper} cells each have characteristic proteins on their surfaces: the *CD8* protein is present on T_{killer} cells, and the *CD4* protein is present on T_{helper} cells (Figure 3–5). Simple tests have been devised for the CD4 and CD8 proteins, and they can be used to identify and count T_{killer} and T_{helper} lymphocytes.

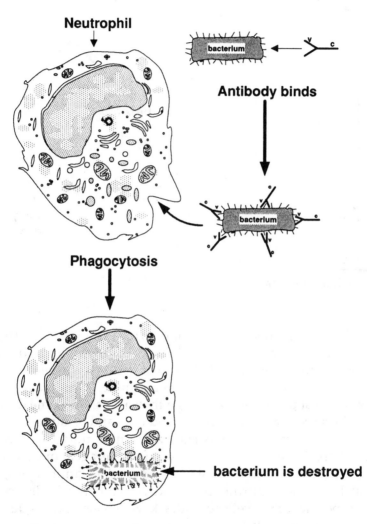
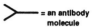

Figure 3–4

The action of phagocytes.

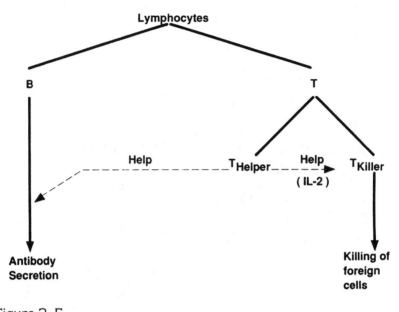

Figure 3–5

Kinds of lymphocytes.

T-lymphocytes get their name from the fact that their maturation depends on passage through the thymus gland. The thymus is a butterfly-shaped gland that lies over the heart.

Natural killer cells are cells that resemble T-lymphocytes in many physical properties, although they also show some differences. These cells attack virus-infected cells and tumor cells and kill them. Natural killer cells exist in normal individuals who have not previously encountered the infectious agent or cancer—this is different from the situation for B- and T-lymphocytes, as we shall see below. Furthermore, individual natural killer cells are not specific for the cells they attack, which also distinguishes them from B- and T-lymphocytes (see below).

THE LYMPHATIC CIRCULATION

Lymphocytes (both B-cells and T-cells) circulate through the blood vessels and also through a second circulatory system, the *lymphatic circulation*. The lymphatic circulation is made up of *lymph channels* in our tissues, which drain lymph fluid from the tissues into structures called *lymph nodes* (Figure 3–6). The lymph nodes contain B-lymphocytes and T-lymphocytes, which can respond to foreign antigens during infections. As an example, suppose a tissue becomes infected with a virus. Pieces of virus or whole virus particles will be transported in the lymph fluid down the lymph channels to the lymph node. In the lymph node, the virus may be recognized as an antigen by B- or T-lymphocytes, which respond by secreting antibodies specific for the virus or producing T-lymphocytes specific for the virus. These antibodies and lymphocytes are then drained from the lymph node through another lymph channel, which joins other lymph channels from other parts of the tissue. Ultimately, fluid from lymph nodes all over the body is collected in a series of lymph vessels that empty into a main vessel called the *thoracic duct*, which empties into the bloodstream. As a result, antibodies and lymphocytes that are produced in response to an infection at one site or tissue will be distributed by the bloodstream throughout the body.

During infections, the lymph nodes near the site of the infection frequently become enlarged. This is because the lymphocytes in these lymph nodes are dividing rapidly and producing large amounts of antibody and cells to fight the infectious agent. You may have noticed swollen glands in your neck if you get a respiratory infection. This is an example of this process.

B-CELLS AND HUMORAL IMMUNITY: THE GENERATION OF ANTIBODIES

Let us now look at how B-lymphocytes respond to a foreign antigen by making antibodies. This part of the immune system is referred to as *humoral immunity*, since it results in production of antibodies which circulate in the bloodstream. *Humor* is derived from the Latin word for fluid.

An antibody molecule is made up of four proteins that are bound together: Two of these proteins are identical and are called *heavy chains*; the other two are also identical and are called *light chains*. A protein is a linear chain of building-block molecules called *amino acids*—much like beads on a string. There are 20 possible amino acids, and the nature of a protein is determined by

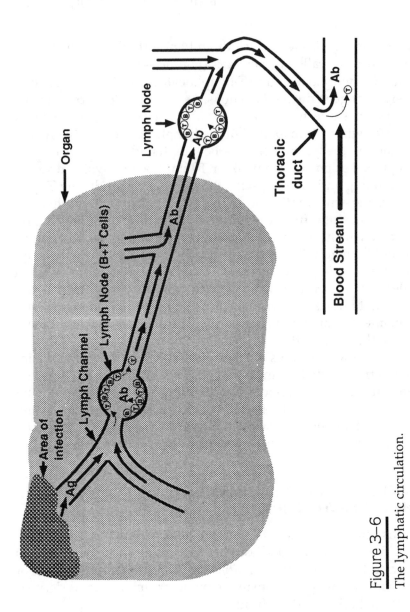

Figure 3–6

The lymphatic circulation.

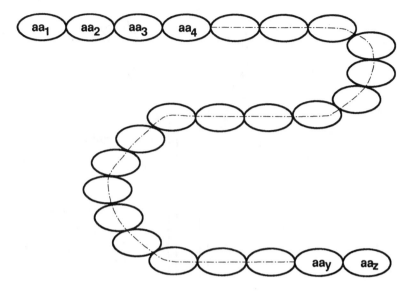

aa$_1$ = amino acid number 1 in the protein chain

aa$_2$ = amino acid number 2 in the protein chain

etc.

Figure 3–7

Protein structure.

the particular sequence of the amino acids it contains (Figure 3–7). In the case of antibodies, the two heavy chain proteins are larger than the two light chain proteins. These proteins are held together by chemical bonding into a Y-shaped molecule, as shown in Figure 3–8. Each antibody molecule is specific for one particular antigen, and this specificity is determined by the sequence of amino acids in the light and heavy chains. If several different antibodies with different specificities are compared, certain regions of the light and heavy chains are very similar for the different antibodies. These regions are referred to as *constant regions* or *C-regions*. Other parts of the light and heavy chain proteins are different for each different antibody in terms of the

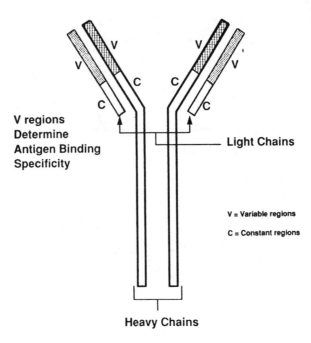

V regions Determine Antigen Binding Specificity

Light Chains

V = Variable regions

C = Constant regions

Heavy Chains

Figure 3–8

Structure of an antibody molecule.

amino acid building-block sequence. These parts are called the *variable regions* or V-regions. The protein sequences of the variable regions determine which antigen the antibody will bind to. An antibody fits its antigen as a key fits only its own lock. Once an antibody is bound to its proper antigen, the C-regions then signal other parts of the immune system to attack—for instance, phagocytosis by a neutrophil or macrophage (Figure 3–4).

One important feature of the humoral immune system is that *each B-lymphocyte makes only one type of antibody,* with a single specificity for an antigen. Thus, each B-lymphocyte is specific for one antigen.

How Does the Immune System Respond to New Antigens?

During our lives, the number of different infectious agents and antigens that we might encounter is infinite. In order to protect us from disease, the immune system must be able to respond to each new antigen upon demand by making new antibodies that recognize it. On the other hand, it is impossible for the immune system to anticipate all possible antigens and continually make all possible antibodies that might be required all the time. This would be much too costly in terms of energy and genetic material. In order to solve this dilemma, the immune system uses two processes: generation of antibody gene diversity by DNA rearrangement, and clonal selection.

Generation of Antibody Gene Diversity by DNA Rearrangement   The genetic information for the antibody proteins is contained within DNA in our chromosomes. *DNA* is a long molecule made up of two strands wound around each other. Each strand is a chain made up of building blocks called *nucleotides,* which contain four possible *bases* (adenine or A, cytosine or C, thymine or T and guanosine or G). The exact order of bases in a DNA molecule specifies the order of amino acid building blocks in the corresponding protein, as shown in Figure 3–9. The sequence of DNA bases that specifies one protein is referred to as

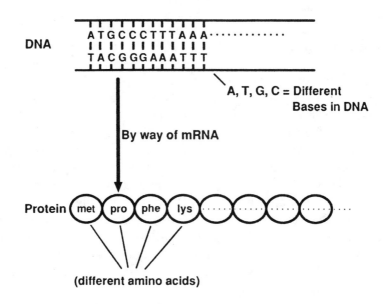

Figure 3–9

How genetic information in DNA is converted into protein.

Before DNA Rearrangement

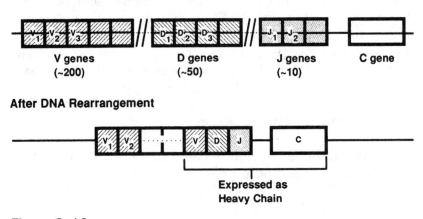

After DNA Rearrangement

Figure 3–10

DNA rearrangement for expression of antibodies.

a *gene*. Each of our chromosomes contains many thousands of genes along its DNA molecule. We inherit two sets of DNA molecules in the form of chromosomes—one set from our mothers and one set from our fathers. The DNA content of most of the cells in the body is the same—different kinds of cells make different kinds of proteins by selecting which genes will be expressed by way of messenger RNA (see Chapter 4) synthesis into protein. However, antibody-producing B-lymphocytes are an exception, at least as far as the region of the chromosome that specifies antibody proteins is concerned.

It is important to remember that each mature B-lymphocyte only produces one kind of antibody. Thus, each B-lymphocyte makes one kind of heavy chain protein and one kind of light chain. All the cells in the body actually contain multiple copies of the genes for variable regions of the heavy and light chain proteins. For the heavy chains, the variable region is actually expressed from three sets of genes called *V-genes*, *D-genes* and *J-genes*. There are about 200 different V-genes, about 50 different D-genes, and about 10 different J-genes. During development and maturation of a B-lymphocyte, the DNA in the chromosomes surrounding the antibody genes is rearranged (Figure 3–10). As a result of the rearrangement, one V-gene is brought together with one D- and one J-gene, and this combination is next to the gene for the constant region. The intervening V, D, and J DNA sequences are deleted. This VDJ combination is expressed along with the constant region gene to give the heavy chain protein. Light chain protein also results from a similar DNA rearrangement process, except that the variable region is specified by only two sets of multiple genes, V-genes and J-genes.

The DNA rearrangements of the antibody genes (VDJ for heavy chain and VJ for light chains) in any individual developing B-lymphocyte are *randomly selected* from the various possible V-, D- and J-genes. Thus, the total number of possible VDJ combinations for the heavy chains in a B-lymphocyte is the *product* of the number of V-genes times the number of D-genes, times the number of J-genes (200 V-genes × 50 D-genes × 10 J-genes = 100,000 combinations for the variable region). Similarly, the total possible VJ combinations for light chain proteins is the product of the number of light chain V-genes times the number of light chain J-genes. Since each B-lymphocyte produces antibody containing one heavy chain and one light chain, the total number of possible antibodies a B-lymphocyte can make is the product of the possible kinds of heavy chain proteins times the possible kinds of light chain proteins. Thus, the number of possible antibodies a B-lymphocyte can make is many millions.

Another process also takes place during B-lymphocyte maturation in addition to the DNA rearrangement of the antibody genes. Individual DNA bases in the genes for the variable regions may be changed or added. These changes will further alter the amino acid sequences of the variable regions for the light and heavy chain proteins. Since these changes also occur on a random basis, they *further increase* the number of kinds of variable regions on the antibody proteins. In practice, the number of possible kinds of antibody proteins that can be made is almost limitless.

Clonal Selection   In a normal, uninfected individual, there are many different B-lymphocytes that have each carried out the DNA rearrangements of their antibody genes, and more mature every day. Initially, these B-lymphocytes express their specific antibodies on their outer surfaces, but they do not secrete antibody and they do not divide. However, if a particular B-lymphocyte recognizes an antigen that binds to its specific antibody (for instance, a protein from an infecting virus), it receives a *signal for activation*. Other B-lymphocytes that are present but that have not bound an antigen do not receive the activation signal. If the B-lymphocyte that has bound an antigen also receives a *second signal* (discussed later), it becomes *fully activated* (Figure 3–11). A fully activated B-lymphocyte does two things: It *divides*

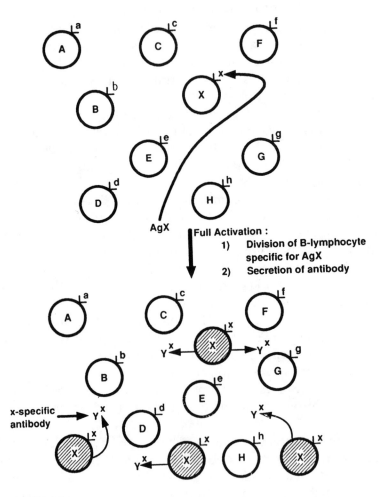

Figure 3–11

Clonal selection of B-lymphocytes.

rapidly and generates more activated B-cells that make the same antibody, and these activated B-cells all *secrete the specific antibody* into the extracellular space (for instance, the lymph or blood). The result of this process is the production of large amounts of antibody specific for the antigen.

The primary immune response   The primary immune response occurs when the immune system encounters an antigen for the first time, as shown in Figure 3–12. For several days after an antigen is encountered, there are no antibodies for the antigen in the bloodstream. This lag period can last for as little as 10 days or as much as several weeks. During the lag period, B-lymphocytes are being primed with antigen and activated to divide and produce antibody. Eventually, antibodies specific for the antigen begin to appear in the bloodstream and increase until they reach a plateau level. Then, if the antigen is eliminated, the antibody level slowly falls until it returns to an undetectable (or barely detectable) level.

In terms of infectious agents such as viruses and bacteria, the lag period during the primary immune response is very important. During this period, no antibodies against the microor-

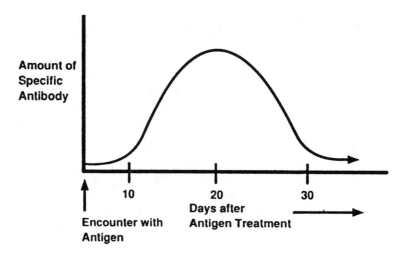

Figure 3–12
_____

The primary immune response.

ganism are being produced. Thus, the individual is susceptible to continued infection during this period—the immune system will begin to fight most efficiently only after antibodies are produced. This window of vulnerability is particularly critical for virus infections, since it is often very difficult to eliminate them once they have become established (see Chapter 4).

During the primary immune response, many different B-lymphocytes become primed and activated to produce antibodies. For instance, in the case of virus infections, B-lymphocytes that make antibodies specific for different virus proteins will be activated. Furthermore, different B-lymphocytes may make antibodies for different parts of a single virus protein. All these B-lymphocytes contribute to the mixture of antibodies that makes up the immune response.

As the primary immune response progresses, the quality of the antibodies also improves. Those antibodies whose variable regions bind most tightly to the antigen become predominant. In addition, the nature of the constant regions of the antibody molecules change. This leads to more efficient signaling by the antibodies to other cells of the immune system (such as phagocytes) for attack and destruction of the foreign cell or microorganism.

The secondary immune response   A secondary immune response occurs in individuals who have previously raised an immunological reaction against a particular antigen—for instance, someone who has recovered from an infection and then later encounters the same infectious agent. In this case, the levels of specific antibodies rise very rapidly, almost without a lag (Figure 3–13). The levels of specific antibody also fall more slowly than after the primary immune response. In addition, the antibodies are the high-quality kind, which bind antigen tightly and efficiently signal to other immune cells for attack. Thus the immune system is said to have *immunological memory*—the ability to respond rapidly and efficiently to an antigen that has been encountered previously.

The nature of the primary and secondary immune responses and immunological memory have led to development of *vaccines* and *vaccination* for controlling infections. The principle is to preexpose an individual to part of an infectious agent, which

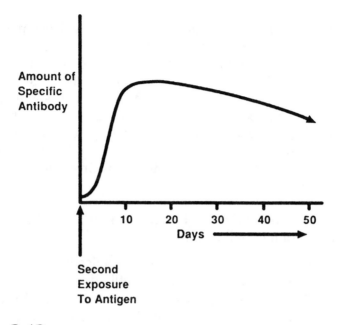

Figure 3–13

The secondary immune response.

cannot cause disease (the vaccine), and to induce production of antibodies against that agent. Repeated injections during the initial immunization are often used to induce the production of high-quality antibodies. After the initial immunization, booster injections at regular intervals stimulate the immunological memory and maintain circulating antibodies for the infectious agent. These antibodies will prevent the infectious agent from establishing themselves in a vaccinated individual.

Tolerance Normal tissues in our bodies contain many molecules that could possibly serve as antigens for our own immune systems. It would be very detrimental to our health if our immune systems attacked our own tissues. Indeed, there are immunological disorders called *autoimmune diseases* that consist of immunological attack by an individual's own tissue (for instance, rheumatoid arthritis). In normal individuals, the immune system distinguishes between *self* and *non-self*. This is achieved by the development of *tolerance* toward normal tissues. For the most part, this is accomplished by elimination during early development of B- and T-lymphocytes that recognize normal tissues. Since these self-specific lymphocytes are absent, no immunological response toward normal tissue will occur. In addition, there are other T-lymphocytes that provide a second line of defense, should some self-specific lymphocytes avoid elimination. These lymphocytes are called $T_{suppressor}$ lymphocytes, and they prevent B-lymphoctes or T_{helper} lymphocytes specific for self- antigens from maturing. $T_{suppressor}$ lymphocytes have CD8 protein on their surfaces, like T_{killer} lymphocytes.

A summary of the humoral immune system To summarize the humoral immune system:

1. B-lymphocytes make antibody molecules, and each B-cell makes only one kind of antibody.
2. The immune response is based on (a) generation of many B-lymphocytes with different antibody specificities by DNA rearrangement and mutation within the antibody genes, and (b) clonal expansion of B-cells that recognize their specific antigen when infection occurs.
3. Antibodies fight infections by (a) direct neutralization of viruses, (b) binding to targets and signaling phagocytes or other white blood cells to attack, or (c) binding to target cells and signaling for other host defense mechanisms.

T-CELLS AND CELL-MEDIATED IMMUNITY

As described above, T-cells make *T-cell antigen receptors* that resemble antibodies made by B-cells. As with an antibody, the T-cell receptor variable region determines its specificity toward an antigen. Also like B-lymphocytes, each T-lymphocyte makes only one kind of T-cell antigen receptor. Thus, each T-lymphocyte is specific for a particular antigen. As described above, T-lymphocytes do not release their receptors; instead, the receptors are anchored in the cell surface, with the variable regions projecting outside. As a result, T-lymphocytes will bind to cells expressing antigen by way of their T-cell antigen receptor. T-lymphocytes represent *cell-medi-*

ated immunity, since the cells themselves specifically bind with antigens. This contrasts with humoral immunity, in which antibodies released from B-lymphocytes carry out the antigen binding.

T_{killer} **lymphocytes** T_{killer} lymphocytes bind cells carrying a foreign antigen and directly kill those cells. Once they have carried out this killing, they release from the target cell, which has been destroyed, and can bind and kill other cells. An example of such an interaction is shown in Figure 3–14. Some examples of cells that T_{killer} cells attack include:

1. *Virus-infected cells.* Most cells infected with viruses express some of the viral proteins on their outer surfaces.

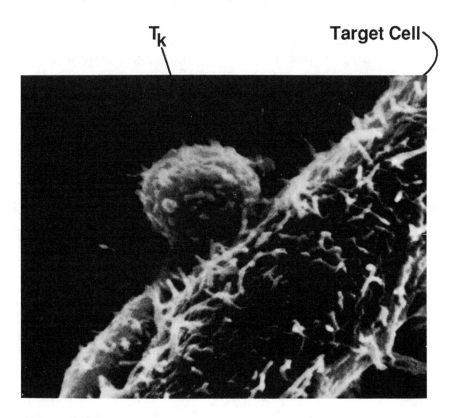

Figure 3–14

T_{killer} lymphocyte killing a target cell (electron microscope picture).

These viral proteins can be recognized as foreign antigens and bind T_{killer} lymphocytes. As a result, the virus-infected cells will be killed.

2. *Tumor cells.* When cancers develop, they often express abnormal proteins on their outer surfaces. These abnormal proteins can also provoke an immune response by T-lymphocytes, which results in immunological attack on the tumor cells. In fact, the immune system is an important part of our natural defense against cancer. During our lives, probably many cells in our bodies begin to develop into tumors, but the cell-mediated immune system eliminates them before they can grow very much. This is called *immunological surveillance*. This is also important in AIDS because, as we shall see, failure of the immune system can result in development of cancers. In addition to T-lymphocytes, natural killer cells (discussed above) are also very important in immunological surveillance.

3. *Tissue Rejection.* When tissue from an unrelated individual is introduced into another person, the cell-mediated immune system will generally raise a strong response and kill the transplanted tissue. This is because cell surface proteins called *histocompatibility antigens* generally differ from individual to individual. This is a major problem for medical procedures such as skin grafting and organ transplantation. If tissue with different histocompatibility antigens is transplanted into an individual, a strong cell-mediated immune response against these antigens will occur, and the transplanted tissue will be destroyed. In the case of organ transplantation, donors and recipients must be carefully matched for histocompatibility antigens in order to avoid rejection of the donor organ. Even then, the recipients must take immunosuppressive drugs permanently to avoid rejection of the donated organ.

T_{helper} **lymphocytes** T_{helper} lymphocytes play a central role in both humoral and cell-mediated immunity. In *humoral immunity*, they provide the second signal necessary for a B-lymphocyte that has bound antigen to divide and secrete antibodies (Figure 3–11). In fact, in order for a B-lymphocyte that has bound antigen to become fully activated, a T_{helper} lymphocyte with the *same antigenic specificity* must bind the antigen as well, as shown in Figure 3–15. Once the specific T_{helper} lymphocyte is bound to the B-lymphocyte by way of the antigen, it provides growth and maturation signals to the B-cell, leading to growth and antibody production. If a T_{helper} lymphocyte of the same antigen specificity as the B-lymphocyte is absent, the B-lymphocyte will not complete maturation, even if it has bound antigen.

T_{helper} cells also play an important role in *cell-mediated* immunity. When T-lymphocytes (either T_{helper} or T_{killer}) bind antigen, they become activated to divide. This will result in increased

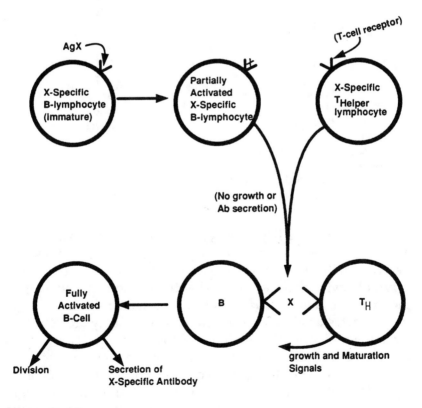

Figure 3–15

The role of T_{helper} cells in B-lymphocyte activation.

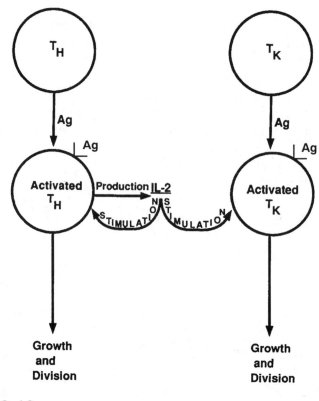

Figure 3–16

T_{helper} cells in cell-mediated immunity.

numbers of specific T-lymphocytes to fight the foreign infectious agent. However, as for many blood cells, T-lymphocytes also need a growth factor in order to divide (as discussed above). For T-lymphocytes that have bound antigen, the required growth factor is one called *interleukin 2* or *IL-2*. It turns out that T_{helper} lymphocytes produce and secrete IL-2 when they are activated by antigen binding (Figure 3–16). Thus, the T_{helper} lymphocytes can stimulate themselves to divide after they bind antigen. On the other hand, most T_{killer} cells do not produce IL-2 even after they bind antigen. They generally rely on IL-2 secreted by neighboring T_{helper} cells in order to divide. In this case, the neighboring T_{helper} cell that produces the IL-2 does not have to be specific for

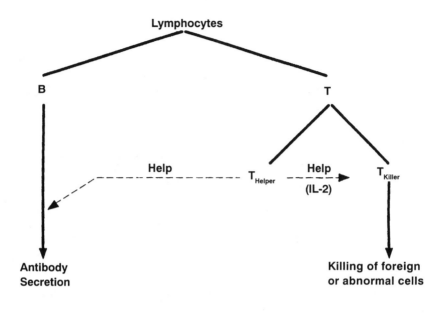

Figure 3–17

The central role of T_{helper} lymphocytes.

the same antigen as the T_{killer} cell it helps. Thus, if T_{helper} lymphocytes are absent, T_{killer} cells cannot divide even if they have bound their specific antigens.

In summary, T_{helper} lymphocytes play a central role in both humoral and cell-mediated immunity, as illustrated in Figure 3–17. As we shall see in the next chapter, the major problem in AIDS is that the causative agent HIV specifically infects and kills T_{helper} lymphocytes. This will cause a failure of both the humoral immune system and cell-mediated immunity. As a result, there will be impaired immunological protection against infectious agents or development of cancer.

Chapter 4

Virology and Human Immunodeficiency Virus

A GENERAL INTRODUCTION TO VIRUSES

- What Are Viruses?
- How Does a Virus Infect a Host?
- A Typical Virus Infection Cycle
- How Do We Treat Viral Infections?

THE LIFE CYCLE OF A RETROVIRUS

THE AIDS VIRUS: HIV

- The Effects of HIV Infection in Individuals
- The HIV Antibody Test
- Potential Problems with the HIV Antibody Test
- How Does HIV Evade the Immune System?

AZT, AN EFFECTIVE THERAPEUTIC AGENT IN AIDS

- Limitations of AZT

WHERE DID HIV COME FROM?

In this chapter, we shall first look at viruses in general, then retroviruses, and then HIV, the virus that causes AIDS, in particular. We will also see how the HIV antibody test (used for screening for HIV infection) works and what it tells us. We will then consider the basis of action of the drug azidothymidine (AZT), which is currently the accepted antiviral treatment for HIV infection.

A GENERAL INTRODUCTION TO VIRUSES

Let's first consider viruses in a general sense. There are many different kinds of viruses, many of which cause disease. Individual viruses may differ in their exact compositions and mechanisms for growth, but all viruses have some properties in common.

What Are Viruses?

Viruses are among the simplest life forms. Here are some of the common features of viruses:

1. *Viruses are obligate intracellular parasites.* This means that viruses cannot replicate and make more of themselves outside of cells. In fact, a pure preparation of virus particles will not grow. In the case of humans, this means that viruses must replicate in some tissue or cell type in our bodies.

7

Condos, PUDs, and Townhouses

C ondominiums (condos), planned unit developments (PUDs), and townhouses are forms of ownership that combine private ownership with joint ownership. They gained popularity in the 1970s and 1980s due to land scarcity, high one-family house prices, and changing life style.

CONDOMINIUMS

Most condominiums consist of an apartment in a new or old multistory building. However, a condo may be a unit in a block of townhouses or a PUD.

When you buy a condominium, you receive a deed conveying fee simple ownership to: (1) the apartment or unit you contracted for and (2) a percentage of the common elements.

A condominium may be owned by the entirety, in severalty, as joint tenants, or tenants in common. As a condominium owner, you receive a separate tax bill. You can sell, mortgage, will, lease, or leave to heirs the apartment you own. If you default on taxes or mortgage payments, your apartment may be sold in foreclosure proceedings that will have no effect on other unit owners.

The Living Unit

In a condominium, the living unit consists of an air lot. It includes the air space and most of the structure within the outer walls and the floor and ceiling of your apartment. For example, the air lot does not include the outer walls, but does include the plaster or sheetrock as well as the paint or wallpaper covering the walls. This is because the outer walls are common elements. Similarly, an air lot does not include the floor, but does include the carpet or tiles installed on it. This is because the floor of one apartment is the ceiling of the apartment below, which means it is a common element.

Air Lot Description. An air lot can be described by one or more of the following three methods:

1. A land survey showing the land and the location of the building. Attached to the land survey is a space survey describing the exact location, inside dimensions, and the floor and ceiling elevations of each apartment.
2. A land survey as described above and architectural drawings, one for each floor showing the floor's height and the location and dimensions of each apartment.
3. A plat of subdivision consisting of drawings in which each air lot is given a number.

The Common Elements

The common elements include the land, exterior of the building, private roads, driveways, sidewalks, lawns, landscaping, stairwells, elevators, hallways, basements, air rights, subsurface rights, and recreational facilities such as a swimming pool, tennis court, and game room, if any. Each owner has easement rights to use the common elements. No owner has the right to partition the common elements.

Some common elements may be located within the individual apartments. For example, the columns that support the floors above are common elements, even though they are located within the boundaries of an apartment. The owners above have an easement of support in these columns. The owner of the apartment cannot tamper with the columns, otherwise the floors above may collapse.

Similarly, the heating and air conditioning ducts, plumbing pipes, and electric wires that pass through one apartment to serve other apartments are common elements. These are included in the declaration (described below) as easements so that no owner should block them.

Condominium Documents

Condominiums are regulated by state laws. In order to establish a property as a condominium, the following documents must be filed with state authorities: (1) the declaration, (2) the bylaws, (3) the rules and regulations, and (4) the plat and architectural drawings.

These documents are substantial. Therefore, you should take the time to familiarize yourself with their contents before making an offer. If you do not understand any provisions or clauses in the documents, ask your lawyer to explain them to you.

Declaration. The word declaration is short *for declaration of covenants, restrictions, easements, and liens.* In some states it is called the *master deed.* It is the principal document that describes the entire project, each apartment, the common elements, the limited common elements (for example, parking spaces) and the units they are assigned to. The declaration further includes:

1. The name of the condominium project.
2. The percentage share of each unit in the undivided ownership of the common elements.
3. The establishment of the bylaws.
4. The establishment of the homeowners association, and the voting rights of each owner.
5. The process of estimating and collecting the assessments, or maintenance fees.
6. The procedures to be followed if an owner doesn't pay his or her maintenance fees.
7. The procedures of amending the declaration.

The Bylaws. The bylaws are the laws that govern the condominium. They are established by the developer at the time of creating the condominium. However, they can be changed or amended by the homeowners association by a majority vote described in the declaration.

Generally, the bylaws include the procedures of electing the board of managers and the board's officers; their authorities and duties; and the duration of their term. They also include the procedures that must be followed in preparing the annual budget for operating and maintaining the common elements and in presenting them to the owners.

Rules and Regulations. Each condominium has a set of rules and regulations that are binding to unit owners. The rules must be reasonable and for the benefit of all unit owners. Furthermore, they should not violate any laws, particularly with respect to discrimination.

The rules may exclude pets or cloth washing machines from individual units, restrict exterior painting to a specific color, or state that the windows be of specific styles and sizes.

Plat and Drawings. The recorded plat and architectural drawings contain the layout of the entire condominium project as well as the number, location and dimensions of each unit. They are a quick means of locating each apartment.

Homeowners Association

The condominium is administered by the homeowners (or condominium owners) association to which every unit owner is automatically a member. When an owner sells his or her unit or dies, his or her membership passes automatically to the purchaser or the owner's heirs. The voting power of each unit owner is usually proportional to his or her ownership to the common elements, unless state laws indicate otherwise.

Board of Managers. The members of the homeowners association elect the board of managers (also called the board of directors) to manage the condominium project. The board may self-manage the condominium project or hire professionals to manage it, depending on the size of the project. The powers, functions, and rights of the board of managers include:

1. Maintaining and repairing the common elements.
2. Calculating the monthly assessments that each owner must pay to cover the costs of operating, maintaining, and insuring the common elements.
3. Establishing a reserve to meet unforeseen expenses, such as frozen pipes or broken heating systems.
4. Establishing the right to access any unit to maintain or repair the common elements or in case of emergency.

Assessments. Assessments, also called *maintenance fees* or *owners assessments,* are the monthly payments that each unit owner makes to pay for operating and maintaining the common elements. These fees are not tax deductible. Furthermore, lenders include them in the cost of housing when they calculate the maximum mortgage loan for which a borrower qualifies.

Each owner is obligated to pay his or her maintenance fee on time. Generally, unpaid maintenance fees become a lien against the apartment. The lien can be enforced by foreclosure proceedings. In some states, the delinquent owner may be evicted from the apartment as if he were a tenant.

The Budget. One of the more important documents you should inspect when buying a condominium is its budget for the past several years. It can tell you a lot about the way the condominium has been financially managed. If the maintenance fees have been rising at a fast rate, it is an indication that the board is not keeping a lid on expenditure. If, on the other hand, the fees have not increased in the past few years, it may be an indication that the board is neglecting the common elements.

Shopping for a Condominium

When shopping for a condominium, ask what is and what is not included in the assessments. In some condominiums there may be additional yearly assessments for heating costs or insurance. Also, you should know if using the recreational facilities is included in the assessments.

One sure way of getting a feeling of the condition of a condominium is to talk to current owners. Ask them if they are satisfied or if they have complaints. Also, meet the board of managers and the secretary of the board. Discuss the budget with the secretary and ask him or her if there are enough reserves to meet emergencies. Also, ask if there are any limitations on the sale or rental of the condominium or if the apartment is subject to right of first refusal (Chapter 9).

In new condominiums, some developers may show that the maintenance fees are less than what they really are or that the project has a sizable reserve only to then withdraw the reserves before handing the condominium to the homeowners association. These acts are illegal.

Condominium Financing

As stated previously, a condominium owner may mortgage his or her fee simple ownership of the apartment and the percentage of the common elements. However, lenders are aware that in addition to mortgage payments, condominium owners must pay monthly assessments. If not paid on time these assessments can become a lien that may be superior to the mortgage. The apartment may be foreclosed upon to satisfy the unpaid assessments.

Also, before making a mortgage loan to a condominium, the lender must examine all the documents that were used in creating the project. The lender knows that the homeowners association can vote to change the percentage of ownership that each owner has in the common elements and to terminate the condominium project.

To protect the interest of lenders, the FNMA/FHLMC uniform mortgage form contains several paragraphs stating the obligations of a condominium borrower towards the lender (Chapter 11).

Timesharing Condominiums

Timesharing condominiums are popular in vacation and resort areas where exclusive ownership of the apartment is not economical. A unit in a timesharing condominium represents a specific time slot of the year, for example, the first 15 days in August or the last 16 days in January. In some arrangements, unit owners are given a different time slot each year.

You may purchase more than one unit. Usually, the buyer receives a deed conveying a fee simple for the duration of his or her time slot.

In addition to the purchase price, the buyer is required to pay yearly maintenance fees to cover the costs of operating, maintaining, and cleaning the common elements and the individual units.

If an owner cannot use the unit in his or her allotted slot, he or she may swap it with another owner or rent it through the manager of the building. An owner may join an international club, if available, where members may swap their slot with a comparable slot at another location in another country. However, there are annual dues for such memberships.

PLANNED UNIT DEVELOPMENTS (PUDs)

A planned unit development (PUD), also called *cluster housing,* is a development that may include assorted types of dwellings (one-family houses, townhouses, etc.) arranged in groups or clusters surrounded by common areas that can be used by all PUD unit owners. The common areas are managed by the homeowners association. Usually, the owner of each unit receives a fee simple to his or her unit and a small piece of private land around it in addition to a percentage of undivided ownership of the common areas. Each owner has easement rights to use the common areas.

The PUD arrangement allows the construction of more units per acre than is permitted in an ordinary subdivision. This results in a lower price per unit. The owner does less site work, which is convenient for working couples and the elderly. It also benefits the local government in that some interior roads are registered as private, which means they will be maintained by the homeowners association.

Before a PUD project starts, the developer must obtain a special permit, or rezoning, from the local government. After a special permit is granted, the developer prepares and submits for recording a set of documents similar to those of a condominium. The documents should show which interior roads are private and which are public.

A PUD unit owner can mortgage his or her fee simple ownership in a manner similar to that of a townhouse or condominium. Generally, financing a PUD is easier than financing a condominium because the owner has a fee simple to land. To protect lenders, the FNMA/FHLMC mortgage form contains several paragraphs stating the obligations of a PUD borrower to the lender (Chapter 11).

Maintenance Assessments. Similar to a condominium, the common areas are owned by the homeowners association, which consists of all unit owners. The association establishes the maintenance assessments that each owner must pay to cover the costs of operating and maintaining the common areas. (These assessments are in addition to mortgage payments.) Delinquent owners may have their units foreclosed upon by the association.

TOWNHOUSES

The word townhouse, also called *row house* in some parts of the country, brings to mind rows of two- to four-story buildings that are almost identical in architectural style and size. Adjoining houses have a common party wall that serves as an exterior wall to both houses. This saves land, construction, and energy costs because the party wall is not exposed to the elements. One disadvantage of row houses is that the party wall has no windows.

Townhouse Ownership

Many townhouses are built in rows that face the street. There are no common elements because each unit can be completely independent of the neighboring units, with the exception of the party walls. The owner of one townhouse owns the lot and the house and improvements on it in fee simple. Additionally, he or she owns the half of the party walls that are constructed on his or her lot, and has an easement of support on the other half of the walls.

Nowadays, townhouses are built in rows perpendicular to the street or in clusters. In such developments, there are common elements such as driveways, water and sewer pipes, electric wires, cable television lines, telephone lines, lawns, landscaping, etc. The common elements, and the creation of a homeowners association to operate and manage them must be stated in a recorded declaration similar to that of a condominium or PUD. To pay for the maintenance and operation of the common elements, townhouse owners are required to pay monthly assessments. These assessments are in addition to mortgage payments.

The land, the boundaries of each house, and the common elements may be shown in a recorded plat of subdivision or in a drawing attached

The structure of a retrovirus is shown in Figure 4–4. The genetic information of a retrovirus is *RNA*. This RNA is covered with a viral *protein coat*; together, the viral RNA and protein coat make up a *core particle*. The core particle also contains several virus-specified enzymes. The core particle is surrounded by a viral *envelope*, which contains membrane lipids and viral envelope protein.

It is important to discuss the *central dogma for genetic information flow* in cells. The central dogma states that genetic information flows in this direction:

$$\text{DNA} \rightarrow \text{RNA} \rightarrow \text{Protein}$$

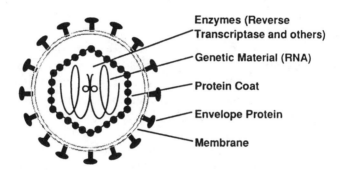

The RNA Genetic Material

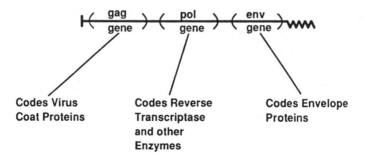

Figure 4–4

The structure of a retrovirus.

That is, the genetic information is carried in *DNA* as a sequence of nucleotide bases (see Figure 3–9). In higher organisms, the DNA is organized into chromosomes that are located in the *nucleus* of the cell. When a gene is expressed, the information from the DNA base sequence is copied or transferred (transcribed) to a related molecule called *RNA* using the DNA molecule as a pattern. The RNA (which is called *messenger RNA* or *mRNA*) then moves from the cell nucleus to the *cytoplasm*. Once in the cytoplasm, the messenger RNA is used as a blueprint for the formation of *proteins* (translation). The proteins then carry out most of the important functions for the cell.

The life cycle of a retrovirus is shown in Figure 4–5. The retrovirus first binds to the surface of an uninfected cell by recognizing a cell receptor. After binding, the virus particle is brought into the cytoplasm of the cell. During this process, the viral envelope is removed, leaving the core particle. Once this happens, a unique virus-specified enzyme called *reverse transcriptase* is activated. This enzyme reads the viral RNA and *makes viral DNA*. The host cell lacks such an enzyme. The viral DNA then moves to the nucleus of the cell, where it is incorporated (or *integrated*) into the host cell's DNA in the chromosomes. Once this viral DNA is integrated into the chromosome, it resembles any other cell gene. As a result, the normal cell machinery reads the integrated viral DNA to make more copies of viral RNA. This viral RNA is then used for *two purposes*: (1) Some of the viral RNA moves to the cytoplasm and functions as *viral messenger RNA* to program the formation of *viral proteins,* and (2) the rest of the viral RNA becomes *genetic material* for new virus particles by moving to the cytoplasm and combining with viral proteins. These virus particles are formed at the cell surface and leave the cell by a process called *budding*.

There are several important characteristics of the retrovirus life cycle. First, most retroviruses do not kill the cells they infect. Second, the fact that these viruses integrate their DNA into host chromosomes allows them to establish a stable carrier state within the infected cell. As a result, once cells are infected with most retroviruses, they will continually produce virus without dying. For some retroviruses, a latent state may also be established, in which the retroviral DNA is integrated

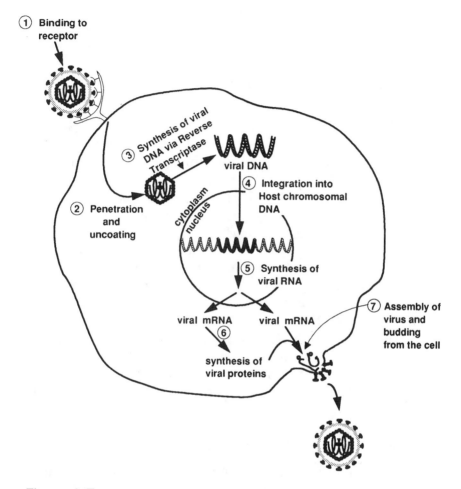

Figure 4–5

The life cycle of a retrovirus.

into the host chromosomes, but it does not program formation of new virus particles. However, at a later time (sometimes years later), the latent viral DNA may become activated by some means, and virus will be produced. This latency process is probably important in AIDS. The viral enzyme *reverse transcriptase* carries out an unusual process in converting the viral RNA genetic information into DNA. This is the *reverse* of genetic information flow according to the central dogma of molecular biology, and this is the reason the enzyme is called reverse transcriptase. This is also where retroviruses get their name—*retro* is from the Latin word for reverse.

All retroviruses have three genes (see Figure 4–4). These genes code for:

1. *Coat proteins that make up the inner virus (core) particle.* The virus gene that specifies these proteins is called the *gag* gene. For HIV, there are three *gag* proteins, p17, p24, and p15.

2. *The enzyme reverse transcriptase, as well as some other enzymes used in virus replication.* The gene that codes these enzymes is the *pol* gene. The other viral enzymes specified by the *pol* gene are *protease* and *integrase*. Protease is involved in maturation of viral proteins as the virus particles bud from the cell, and integrase is responsible for integration of the viral DNA into the cell's chromosomal DNA.

3. *The proteins of the viral envelope.* The gene that codes for these proteins is the *env* gene. A protein coded by the *env* gene is responsible for binding the virus to the cell receptor. For HIV, there are two *env* proteins, gp120 and gp41.

THE AIDS VIRUS: HIV

The virus that causes AIDS is Human Immunodeficiency Virus (HIV) (Figure 4–6). Other names that have been used previously for HIV include HTLV-III, LAV, and ARV. HIV belongs to a subgroup of retroviruses called *lentiviruses* (meaning *slow viruses,* since they often cause disease extremely slowly); other lentiviruses have been found in such diverse species as cats, sheep, goats, horses, and monkeys. Actually, the virus responsible for the great majority of AIDS cases in the United States, Europe, and Africa is called HIV-1. A second virus related to HIV-1 has been isolated in Africa: HIV-2 (see Chapter 6). HIV-2 also appears to cause AIDS. In this book, we will refer to the AIDS virus simply as HIV, and this will almost always mean HIV-1.

Several features about the structure and replication of HIV are important (Figure 4–7a):

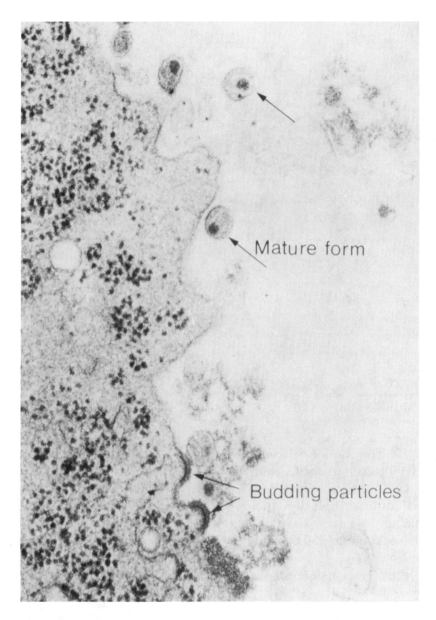

Mature form

Budding particles

Figure 4–6

An electron microscope picture of an HIV-infected cell. The cytoplasm of the cell is on the left, and the exterior of the cell is on the right. Budding HIV particles are indicated, as well as mature virus particles released from the cell. (*Courtesy of the Centers for Disease Control*)

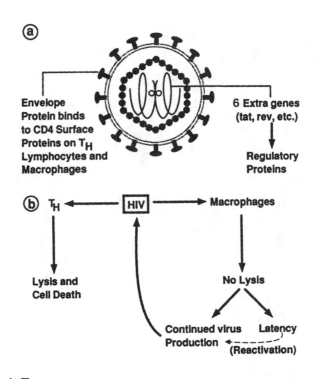

Figure 4–7

Unusual features of HIV.

The nature of the HIV receptor   The cell receptor that HIV binds to is the *CD4 surface protein*. As described in Chapter 2, CD4 protein is present on T_{helper} lymphocytes. In fact, this is the predominant cell type that has CD4 protein. In addition, some macrophages also have CD4 protein. Most other cells in the body do *not* contain CD4 protein. As a result, *the main cells that HIV can infect are T_{helper} lymphocytes and macrophages*. The HIV envelope protein responsible for virus binding to CD4 protein is called gp120.

Extra genes   As all retroviruses do, HIV contains the three genes for coat proteins, reverse transcriptase, and envelope proteins. In addition, HIV contains genes that specify six additional proteins. These are regulatory proteins that give HIV finer levels of control and a more versatile life cycle. Two of the best-known of these genes are *tat*, which is an up-regulator or amplifier of viral gene expression in the infected cell, and *rev*, which shifts the balance from production of viral regulatory proteins to proteins that make up virus particles.

These extra genes may be important in allowing the virus to establish a latent or inactive state in some infected cells, followed by reactivation at later times. The other HIV genes specify proteins called *nef, vpu, vif, and vpx*.

Killing of T$_{helper}$ lymphocytes   In contrast to most retroviral infections, *infection of T$_{helper}$ lymphocytes with HIV results in cell death* (Figure 4–7b). Considering the pivotal role that T$_{helper}$ lymphocytes play in both humoral and cell-mediated immunity (see Chapter 3), it is possible to understand how infection with HIV can ultimately lead to collapse of the immune system.

Nonlytic infection of macrophages   When HIV infects macrophages, it follows a course that is typical of other retroviruses, in that the infected macrophages are not killed (Figure 4–7b). In most cases, the macrophages continue to produce HIV virus particles, while other macrophages establish a latent state of HIV infection. These infected macrophages are an important reservoir of infection in an HIV-infected individual. This may also explain how many years can elapse between the time of initial infection and development of clinical AIDS symptoms.

The Effects of HIV Infection in Individuals

Let's now consider the results of HIV infection at the level of infected people. The routes of HIV infection are covered in Chapters 6 and 7, so here we will start at the time a person becomes infected. There is a detailed description of AIDS as a clinical disease in the next chapter, but an overview is useful at this point.

The progression of events after HIV infection is shown in Figure 4–8. After HIV infection, there are generally very few initial symptoms—perhaps a mild flulike illness or swollen glands. Most individuals then remain free of any clinical symptoms for variable lengths of time—up to many years. Individuals who are HIV infected but who do not show any signs of disease are re-

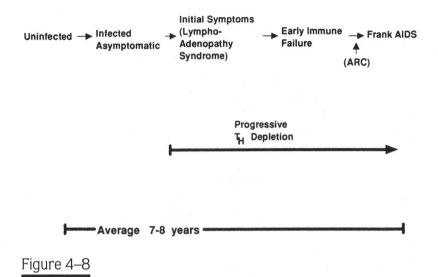

Figure 4–8

Consequences of HIV infection.

ferred to as *asymptomatic*. It is generally difficult to detect infectious HIV virus in infected asymptomatic individuals. Indeed, even as individuals develop clinical symptoms, they generally have rather low levels of infectious HIV. One of the puzzles about HIV is how it can cause such devastating disease with such apparently low levels of circulating virus. During the asymptomatic period, individuals generally produce *antibodies* to HIV. Unfortunately, these antibodies are not sufficient to prevent continued HIV infection as the disease progresses. However, they provide a useful diagnosis for HIV infection, as we shall see below.

As time passes, many HIV-infected individuals begin to experience symptoms of HIV infection. Some initial symptoms include persistent enlarged lymph glands (*lymphoadenopathy syndrome* or *LAS*) and fevers or night sweats. As the disease worsens, a continuum of progressively more serious conditions develops as the immune system weakens, ultimately resulting in full-blown or frank AIDS. During the early periods of the AIDS epidemic, doctors also used a classification called *ARC* or *AIDS-Related Complex*. Individuals were classified as having ARC if they showed fewer of the characteristic opportunistic infections or cancers (see below) than patients with frank AIDS. The term *ARC* is used less frequently today after the progressive nature of HIV infection has become apparent. The progression from asymptomatic infection to AIDS is accompanied by a progressive depletion of T_{helper} lymphocytes by HIV infection. Ultimately, there is a profound lack of T_{helper} lymphocytes, which results in the failure of both humoral and cell-mediated immunity. In individuals with normal immune systems, the T_{helper} counts are typically over 1,000 per cubic millimeter of blood, while in patients with frank AIDS, these may be well under 100 per cubic millimeter.

The clinical manifestations of AIDS are covered in detail in Chapter 5. They can be summarized briefly here.

Opportunistic infections   These are infections by microorganisms that normally do not cause problems in healthy individuals. However, in individuals with weakened immune systems, these microorganisms can take hold and cause devastating infections. One important opportunistic infection is *pneumocystis carinii* (*PCP pneumonia*), caused by a fungus microbe.

Cancers   Cell-mediated immunity also plays an important role in defense against development of cancers (immune surveillance—see Chapter 3). HIV-infected individuals develop several cancers with very high frequency. One example of an AIDS-related cancer is *Kaposi's sarcoma.*

Weight loss   Many AIDS patients suffer from profound weight loss or wasting. The mechanism for this is not yet understood.

Mental impairment   HIV can also establish infection in the nervous system. This can result in muscle spasms or tics. More serious is infection of the central nervous system, which can result in *AIDS-related dementia,* in which individuals lose the ability to reason.

Individual AIDS patients may suffer from one or more of these manifestations. Indeed, recurrent bouts with different opportunistic infections or cancers may be experienced.

Since the major problem in AIDS is a loss of T_{helper} lymphocyte function, monitoring of the numbers of T_{helper} lymphocytes is important in clinical monitoring of HIV-infected individuals. Doctors can perform a test for these cells, and the results are reported in terms of T_{helper} (or T4 or CD4) lymphocyte numbers. A few years ago, the tests were frequently reported as the ratio of T_{helper} to T_{killer} lymphocytes in the blood (also T4/T8 or helper-to-suppressor ratios). An inversion of the normal T_{helper}/T_{killer} lymphocyte ratio is often an early sign of HIV infection.

The likelihood that an HIV-infected individual will develop full-blown AIDS is discussed in more detail in Chapter 6. Current estimates are that more than 70 percent of HIV-infected individuals will develop AIDS with an average time to disease of eight or more years.

One of the enigmas of HIV infection and AIDS was the fact that, until the disease has progressed quite far, there is actually very little infectious HIV apparent in the blood of an infected individual. This fact has even led some people to question whether HIV is the cause of AIDS, although the epidemiological and clinical results make it very clear that this is the case. However, very recent studies with advanced techniques have shown that there is extensive infection of T-lymphocytes in lymph nodes, although the infected cells are not released into the bloodstream until late in the disease.

The HIV Antibody Test

Within a year of the isolation of HIV as the causative agent of AIDS, a test was developed that determines if an individual has been exposed to HIV. The procedure is to test whether an individual has antibodies to HIV virus proteins. These antibodies appear in those who have been previously infected with HIV and have made antibodies against the virus (see Chapter 3).

The most common HIV antibody test is called an *ELISA* test, shown in Figure 4–9. In an ELISA assay, virus protein is first attached to a small laboratory dish. A serum sample is prepared from the blood of the individual to be tested, and it is placed in the dish containing bound HIV viral proteins. If HIV-specific antibodies are present in the serum, they will become tightly bound

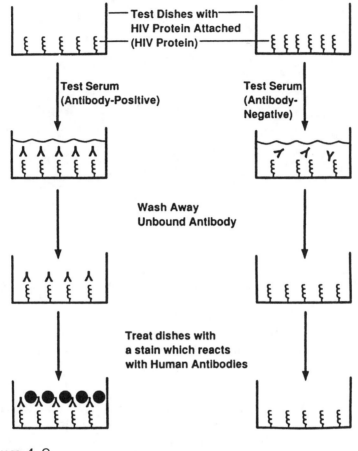

Figure 4–9

The ELISA test for HIV antibody.

to the dish by way of the HIV proteins. The serum is then re-moved, and the dish is washed—during this procedure, only antibodies specific for HIV will be retained. The dish is then re-acted with a stain that will detect *any* human antibodies. Thus, dishes that were exposed to serum containing HIV-specific anti-bodies will be stained, while dishes from antibody-negative se-rum samples will be unstained. This procedure has been automated, so that many blood samples can be tested at once (Figure 4–10). The current ELISA tests are better than 99.9 per-

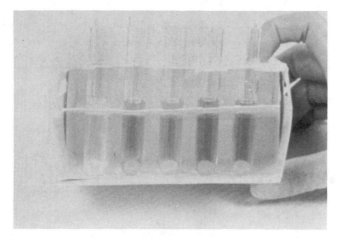

Figure 4–10

A modified ELISA test is shown. In this case, the virus proteins are attached to small beads that can float in solution, instead of the bottom of the dish. The tube on the left shows a test of a blood sample that does not have HIV-specific antibodies. The four tubes on the right show test of HIV antibody-positive blood samples. The color in the tubes on the right indicates the presence of HIV antibodies. (*Courtesy of Abbot Laboratories, Diagnostic Division*)

cent accurate. That is, fewer than 0.1 percent of HIV-negative individuals incorrectly score as positive by the ELISA test. Likewise, fewer than 0.1 percent of HIV antibody-positive serum samples are missed by the test.

Potential Problems with the HIV Antibody Test

Although this test has been extremely important in furthering our knowledge of how the virus spreads and causes disease, there are several potential problems with it.

False positives These are individuals who are not HIV-infected but who test antibody-positive in the ELISA assay. Clearly, this can be an extremely frightening experience. With current ELISA assays, the frequency of false positives is less than 1 in 1,000 (0.1 percent) uninfected individuals. False positives are a particular problem if populations with low frequencies of HIV infection are tested. In these cases, a high proportion of the individuals who score positive could be false positives. This is one of the arguments (besides cost) against routine HIV antibody screening of the general U.S. population, where current prevalences of infection are less than 1 percent—many of the individuals identified as antibody positive in such a mass screening could actually be false positives.

Because of the significant false positive rate for the ELISA test, a second, more specific test for HIV antibodies is also used: the *Western blot* test. This technique has a lower incidence of false positives than the ELISA assay. In practice, serum samples that score antibody positive by the ELISA test are generally retested by the Western blot procedure. Serum samples are considered positive if they are found to contain HIV-specific antibodies by both tests. New and improved tests (more sensitive and/or more accurate) for HIV infection are currently undergoing development.

False negatives   A more important problem is individuals who are infected with HIV but who do not score positive in the HIV antibody test. Such individuals fall into two categories:

1. *Recently infected individuals.* As was discussed in Chapter 3, the immune system has a lag period between initial exposure to an antigen and the production of antibodies. In the case of HIV infection, this lag can range up to six months or longer. Thus, individuals who have been recently infected with HIV will not score positive in the antibody test.

2. *Infected individuals who never mount an immune response.* Since the immune response varies from person to person, a few infected individuals do not produce antibodies to HIV. There are rare but documented cases of individuals who remain antibody negative but spread HIV infection to their sexual partners.

The HIV antibody test measures whether an individual has circulating antibodies to HIV. However, strictly speaking, the test does *not* indicate if an antibody-positive individual still harbors infectious virus. Some individuals who are exposed to HIV might have raised a successful immune response and completely eliminated the infection. However, by and large, most HIV-antibody positive individuals turn out to be still infected.

While the HIV antibody test is the routine test used to identify individuals who have been exposed to HIV, other tests for viral infection are used as well. In particular, it is advantageous to know the amount of circulating virus particles in an infected individual, since the levels of virus are generally low, but they frequently rise when frank AIDS develops. The most common test for virus particles is to measure the level of the major HIV core protein (p24 protein) in the blood. Because this test detects p24 protein by use of an antibody against it, it is sometimes referred to as a test for p24 antigen.

More sensitive tests for HIV infection are under development. This is important because in an HIV-infected individual, most cells are not infected—even among CD4-positive T_H lymphocytes and monocytes/macrophages. A newly developed technique called *polymerase chain reaction* or PCR has been developed; it tests for HIV DNA in infected cells. The PCR test can detect as few as one HIV-infected cell among a million uninfected ones and is currently being used in research laboratories.

How Does HIV Evade the Immune System?

One of the paradoxes about HIV infection is that most infected individuals contain HIV antibodies, but the disease eventually occurs in most cases, even in the presence of these antibodies. This means that HIV antibodies are unable to prevent onset of AIDS. This may be due to several factors. First, the levels of antibodies raised might be insufficient to block the spread of infectious virus. In addition, antibodies can be produced against different parts of the virus. Only some of these antibodies (*neutralizing antibodies*) can inactivate virus and prevent infection. Finally, several unique features of HIV infection provide the virus with ways to evade the immune system.

High mutation rates   The HIV envelope proteins are on the outside of the virus particle, and they are important in attaching the virus to the cell receptor. As such, they are the most important targets for neutralizing antibodies. HIV has an unusually high mutation rate, estimated as one DNA base mutation each time an HIV DNA molecule is made by reverse transcriptase. The consequence of this is that mutations in the HIV *env* gene occur very frequently, so that the exact amino acid sequence of the envelope proteins changes quite rapidly during successive cycles of infection. Equivalent mutations in the gag and pol genes are not compatible with virus survival. Changes in the makeup of HIV envelope proteins have even been observed over time within the same person. Thus, even though an infected individual may raise neutralizing antibodies to the initial infecting virus, those antibodies may not be able to neutralize subsequent viruses with mutated envelope proteins. Thus, HIV can keep one step ahead of the immune system and continue infection.

Latent states   HIV can establish *latent states* in some cells. In these cells, the viral DNA is maintained, but virus proteins are not expressed. As a result, these latently infected cells will not be recognized or attacked by the immune system but will remain as reservoirs for infectious virus. At later times, the virus may be activated from these cells. Macrophages are probably the major cells that carry latent HIV, since initial HIV infection does not kill them. In addition, T_{helper} cells latently infected with HIV may also exist, although in fewer numbers than latently infected macrophages.

Reactivation of latent HIV from carrier cells may also be important in AIDS progression. Infection of cells carrying latent HIV with certain other viruses, such as herpes simplex or cytomegalovirus, may reactivate the HIV. In addition, other stimuli to the immune system (such as infection with other microorganisms) can result in production of factors that reactivate HIV. These secondary infections may be important cofactors in AIDS progression.

Cell-to-cell spread   HIV can carry out infection by *cell-to-cell spread*. That is, if an HIV-infected cell comes into contact with an uninfected cell, the virus may pass to the uninfected cell directly. Neutralizing antibodies are unable to prevent this process, since they can only attack virus when it is outside cells.

These properties of HIV also pose another problem. Vaccines are our front line of defense against most virus infections, as described earlier in this chapter. However, the ability of HIV to evade the immune system means that it will much more difficult to design an effective anti-HIV vaccine.

AZIDOTHYMIDINE (AZT), AN EFFECTIVE THERAPEUTIC AGENT IN AIDS

The primary drug against HIV infection and AIDS is azidothymidine (or zidovudine, or AZT, or Retrovir). The effectiveness and use of AZT are described more in Chapters 5 and 6. However, let's consider its mode of action here.

Azidothymidine is very similar in chemical structure to thymidine, one of the building blocks of DNA. However, when AZT is incorporated in place of thymidine during the DNA assembly process, its structure aborts further DNA assembly. This inactivates any growing DNA molecule that has incorporated AZT. During HIV infection, if AZT is present, HIV reverse transcriptase will readily incorporate it into the viral DNA. This will inactivate the viral DNA. It is important that the enzymes responsible for making the chromosomal DNA of the cell (cellular DNA polymerases) do *not* efficiently incorporate AZT into DNA. As a result, the cell can continue to grow and make its genetic material, but HIV cannot replicate efficiently. Thus, AZT is a *selective poison* for HIV. It exploits an Achilles heel of the virus— reverse transcriptase. This enzyme plays no role in the uninfected cell, but it is vital to the virus. An agent that affects this enzyme will have no effect on the uninfected cell but will inhibit virus infection. This is shown in Figure 4–11.

Limitations of AZT

While AZT is an effective drug in AIDS treatment, it has some limitations.

Toxic side effects   Normal cellular DNA polymerases do not efficiently incorporate AZT into DNA in comparison to HIV reverse transcriptase—the basis for the drug's selectivity. However, cellular DNA polymerases do incorporate some AZT into cell DNA at low levels. During prolonged treatment, this can

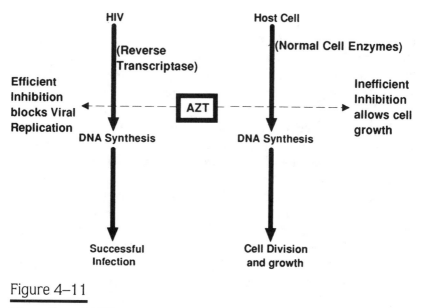

Figure 4–11

The action of AZT.

lead to death of normal cells. Anemia is a common side effect in individuals taking AZT; it results from killing of blood cells by the drug.

Inability to halt progression to AIDS While AZT treatment improves the clinical condition of individuals with frank AIDS and also slows progression of asymptomatic people to AIDS, it is not a cure (see Chapter 5). While the exact reason for the inability of AZT to halt progression to AIDS is not understood, one possibility is that the virus may mutate in the individual. Indeed, AZT-resistant HIV has been detected in individuals who have been taking AZT.

Development of AZT-resistant variants As described above, HIV has a high mutation rate. Normally, few mutations in the *pol* gene appear because they decrease the virus's growth rate if they occur. However, under the selective pressure of AZT, AZT-resistant variants of HIV appear that have mutated reverse transcriptase. This mutated enzyme does not incorporate AZT as efficiently, making the virus less sensitive to the drug. AZT-resistant HIV variants have been detected in AIDS patients who are taking AZT, and it is possible that these variants may contribute to the inability of AZT to prevent the effects of HIV indefinitely. However, the relative importance of AZT-resistant HIV variants in the disease process has not been determined yet.

Despite its limitations, the effectiveness of AZT in treating AIDS patients has a very important implication. Even in individuals who are already infected, *prevention of continued HIV infection improves the clinical status.* Thus, other drugs that selectively inhibit HIV reverse transcriptase are likely to be useful therapeutic agents, particularly if they can overcome some of the limitations of AZT (see Chapter 5). Moreover, the other HIV proteins are all potential Achilles heels for the virus as well. Agents that interfere with the action of any of these proteins may also be useful therapeutic agents. AIDS researchers are devoting a great deal of effort to developing new anti-HIV drugs.

WHERE DID HIV COME FROM?

Molecular biologists have examined the genetic structure of HIV (actually HIV-1 and HIV-2) in great detail and compared it to the structure of other retroviruses of the lentivirus subclass. From these studies, it is clear that HIV shares a common origin with other lentiviruses, and they evolved from a common ancestral retrovirus over millions of years. Epidemiological studies tell us that the HIV that exists today probably evolved to its current form in central Africa hundreds of thousands of years ago. Fifteen to twenty years ago, it spread into high-density populations in Africa and the Western world, leading to the AIDS epidemic. Recent changes in human social behavior, such as the sexual revolution, may have also contributed to the spread of HIV infection.

Numerous apocryphal stories as to the origin of HIV have circulated since the beginning of the AIDS epidemic. These include: HIV was the result of germ warfare research by the CIA; HIV was a laboratory accident involving recombinant DNA; HIV resulted from a plot between Israel and South Africa; HIV resulted from sexual relations between humans and sheep; HIV resulted from sexual relations between humans and monkeys. *None of these are true.*

Chapter 5

Clinical Manifestations of AIDS

EXPOSURE, INFECTION, AND DISEASE

- Exposure versus Infection
- Infection versus Disease

INITIAL INFECTION AND THE ASYMPTOMATAIC PERIOD

- Mononucleosis-like Illness
- Brain Infection (Encephalopathy)

INITIAL DISEASE SYMPTOMS

- Wasting Syndrome
- Lymphadenopathy Syndrome
- Neurological Disease

DAMAGE TO THE IMMUNE SYSTEM AND FRANK AIDS

- Early Immune Failure
- Frank AIDS
  Fungal Infections
  Protozoal Infections
  Bacterial Infections
  Viral Infections
  Cancers

AZT TREATMENT IN AIDS

In the previous two chapters, we learned about AIDS at the cellular and subcellular levels. In particular, cells of the immune system were discussed, and the effects of HIV infection on those cells were presented. With that background, we can now consider the effects of HIV in terms of a whole person—the actual symptoms that infected individuals experience. A brief overview of AIDS at the organismal level is included in Chapter 4, and in this chapter, a detailed description of the clinical manifestations of AIDS is presented. While the physical manifestations of the disease are of great importance to AIDS patients and their health-care providers, it is important to remember the human side of the disease as well. AIDS is often a fatal disease. For persons to learn that they are infected with HIV evokes tremendous emotional stress. Counselors are trained to help a patient deal with this psychologically difficult situation. In this chapter, we will simply present the biological or clinical aspects of AIDS. The psychological consequences of being infected with HIV or learning that one is HIV-infected are at least as important but will be considered elsewhere.

EXPOSURE, INFECTION, AND DISEASE

In terms of AIDS and HIV at the organismal level, it is important to consider interaction of the virus with a susceptible individual. Three important concepts in the interaction are *exposure, infection,* and *disease.*

Exposure versus Infection

When an HIV-infected individual encounters an uninfected person, this does not always result in transmission of HIV to the uninfected person. Indeed, even if exposure occurs by one of the three routes known to transmit the virus (blood, birth, and sex), only a fraction of the exposed people will be infected. The relative risk factors affecting the efficiency of HIV transmission are discussed in Chapters 6 and 7. As we shall see, different kinds of exposure between infected and uninfected individuals have different probabilities of leading to infection.

As introduced in Chapter 4, most individuals who are exposed to HIV and become infected do not show signs of illness right away. Thus, it is generally not possible to distinguish infected and uninfected people simply on the basis of their physical well-being. The HIV antibody test is invaluable in identifying individuals infected with HIV (see Chapter 4). Generally, an infected person will begin to produce antibodies against HIV (*seroconvert*) two to three months after infection, although the time for seroconversion is variable and can last as long as a year or more. In practical terms, someone who was exposed to HIV is generally considered to be uninfected if he or she is seronegative for HIV antibodies six months after the last exposure to HIV and remains seronegative for another six months during which time no other potential exposures occurred.

Infection versus Disease

Even among individuals who become infected with a virus, not necessarily everybody will develop physical symptoms. For many viruses, most of the infected individuals actually never develop physical signs of illness. Unfortunately, most people infected with HIV ultimately develop some disease symptoms (see Chapter 6).

The disease symptoms that result from virus infection are caused by destruction or damage of cells and tissues in the infected person. In some cases, the damage may result from direct killing of cells by the infecting virus. In other cases, the physical symptoms may result from indirect effects of the virus. In the case of AIDS, most of the physical symptoms are the indirect results of damage to the immune system by HIV (see Chapters 3 and 4).

Many virus infections can cause a variety of physical symptoms. Other factors can influence the exact nature of the symptoms in a particular individual, including age, sex, genetic makeup, nutrition, environmental factors, and encounters with other infectious agents. As we shall see, this is particularly true for AIDS, in which the symptoms result from indirect immunological damage.

A schematic diagram of the different clinical stages of HIV infection is shown in Figure 5–1. In time sequence, the stages can be grouped into three categories: (1) *Initial infection and the asymptomatic period,* (2) *initial symptoms,* and (3) *immunological damage* (early signs through frank AIDS).

INITIAL INFECTION AND THE ASYMPTOMATIC PERIOD

Many people who become infected with HIV never experience any symptoms at the time of initial infection. On the other hand, some HIV-infected people do develop some relatively mild disease symptoms right after infection (prior to seroconversion). These are referred to as *acute symptoms,* and they generally last only a few days and then disappear. Two types of acute symptoms can occur.

Mononucleosis-like Illness

The most common early illness seen with HIV infection resembles another viral disease, mononucleosis. Mononucleosis is not exclusive to a particular virus, in that other viral infections can cause these symptoms as well. The most prominent symptoms are swollen lymph glands. In the case of HIV infection, this includes lymph glands throughout the body—called generalized *lymphadenopathy.* In addition, there may also be a sore throat, a fever, and a skin rash. Because these symptoms also result from infection by other viruses, it is not possible to diagnose an HIV infection solely based on the appearance of these symptoms.

Initial Infection

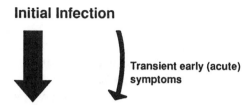

Transient early (acute) symptoms

Asymptomatic

Initial Symptoms

1. Lymphadenopathy

2. Wasting syndrome / Fever / Night sweats

3. Neurological disease

Early immune failure

1. Shingles (VZV)

2. Thrush (Candida)

3. Hairy Leukoplakia (EBV)

Frank AIDS (Opportunistic Infections and Cancers)

1. Pneumonia (Pneumocystis)　　5. Bacterial infection (TB like)

2. Kaposi's sarcoma　　6. Viral infection (CMV)

3. Other protozoan infections　　7. Other cancer (lymphoma)

4. Systemic Fungal infection

Figure 5–1

The progression of symptoms in AIDS. (The above symptoms may be additive.)

Brain Infection (Encephalopathy)

HIV infection of the brain can occur at this early time and lead to brain swelling or inflammation, particularly of the brain lining or meninges. In medical terms, this is called *encephalopathy*. Macrophage cells in the brain appear to be prominent sites for virus replication during this time. The brain inflammation may result from the influx of immune system cells to fight the infection or the release from infected cells of highly active molecules that can affect other brain cells. The brain inflammation causes symptoms of headache and fever. Brain function can be impaired to various degrees. Often the person will have difficulty in concentrating, remembering, or solving problems. There may also be some personality changes during the acute phase.

During the acute phase of infection, significant levels of circulating HIV are generally produced. Following the acute phase, the infected person will usually feel well but become seropositive for HIV. This is referred to as the period of *asymptomatic infection*. Generally, circulating levels of infectious HIV are low during the asymptomatic period. Some infected people will not have detectable infectious HIV in their blood and are *latently* infected (see Chapter 4). In these people, the HIV genetic information is integrated into the chromosomes of macrophages or lymphocytes but is silent. At some later time, however, the HIV genetic information may become activated and begin to produce virus. Most infected people, however, produce low levels of HIV in their blood and are *persistently* or *chronically* infected. As mentioned above, the asymptomatic period may last as long as eight years or more or as little as several months. We do not yet understand why there is such variability.

During the asymptomatic period, some type of balance apparently exists between HIV infection and the immune system in the infected person. Ultimately, for most individuals, changes in the virus or the immune system allow the HIV infection to escape from control and lead to disease.

INITIAL DISEASE SYMPTOMS

The initial disease that follows the asymptomatic period falls into three major classes. An infected person may have symptoms from more than one of these classes.

Wasting Syndrome

The two symptoms seen with this syndrome are a sudden and otherwise unexplained *loss in body weight* (more than 10 percent of total body weight) and *fevers*, usually at night, that cause *night sweats*. The weight loss is usually progressive, leading to wasting away of the infected person, and may be accompanied by diarrhea. This wasting syndrome is very reminiscent of the progressive loss of body weight by cancer patients. The fevers can involve dangerously high temperatures (106–107° Fahrenheit), which can result in brain damage. Normally, the body controls high internal temperatures by sweating. The night sweats result from the bodies of infected individuals attempting to lower their temperatures.

Lymphadenopathy Syndrome

As described above, *lymphadenopathy* means swelling of the lymph glands. Lymphadenopathy sometimes is also an acute symptom of HIV infection, but in lymphadenopathy syndrome (*LAS*), the lymph gland enlargement is persistent. This condition as also called *persistent generalized lymphadenopathy* or *PGL*. In LAS, the lymph glands in the head and neck, the armpits, and the groin are usually swollen, although they generally are not painful. Some infected people will experience both LAS and the wasting syndrome described above. In the past, lymphadenopathy was one of a group of symptoms that was associated with AIDS-related complex (ARC; see Chapter 4), a condition considered less serious than AIDS. However, the term *ARC* is used less frequently nowadays, and lymphadenopathy actually can occur at various different stages of the disease.

Neurological Disease

The HIV infection can spread to the brain and either damage the brain directly or lead to damage by other infectious agents. In addition, other parts of the nervous system can be damaged and cause different neurological symptoms. About one third of all AIDS patients will have some of the following neurological symptoms.

Dementias   When the brain itself is damaged, mental functions are impaired. With HIV infection, this is usually a progressive situation. Initially, this may appear as simple forgetfulness about where things are. As the disease progresses, the loss of mental function can become more serious: The infected person may have difficulty reasoning and performing other mental tasks. Depression, social withdrawal, and personality changes are also common. Eventually, as the disease progresses, infected people may become demented and unable to care for themselves. For some AIDS patients, this progression leads to the patient entering a coma followed by death, if other infections or cancers do not kill the patient first. Death usually occurs several months following the onset of dementia.

Spinal cord damage (myelopathy)   Because the spinal cord transmits nerve impulses to the muscles of the body, damage to the spinal cord can result in weakness or paralysis of voluntary muscles. As a result, HIV infection can lead to spinal cord swelling (*myelopathy*) and paralysis or weakness of the limbs.

Peripheral nerve damage (neuropathy)   Some people infected with HIV will experience swelling (neuropathy) of the peripheral nerves. These nerves are involved in sensing pain. When they are damaged, they can cause burning or stinging sensations, usually in the hands or feet. In addition, the occurrence of numbness, especially in the feet, is frequent.

These initial symptoms of HIV infection are not mutually exclusive. Individual patients may experience a mixture of any of these illnesses.

DAMAGE TO THE IMMUNE SYSTEM AND FRANK AIDS

As described in Chapter 4, the major problem in HIV infection is damage to the immune system. Two major consequences result from immunological damage: the occurrence of *opportunistic infections* caused by infectious agents that are normally held in check by healthy immune systems, and the development of *cancers* that also result from failure of the immune system (see Chapter 3). In HIV-infected individuals, both opportunistic infections and cancers may develop (sometimes at the same time), but opportunistic infections are generally the more common causes of death.

As indicated in Chapter 4, the breakdown of the immune system in HIV-infected individuals is a continuous and gradual process. It generally begins with the occurrence of relatively minor opportunistic infections and usually progresses to severe and life-threatening disease—frank AIDS. After the isolation of HIV, an early medical definition for diagnosing AIDS was evidence of HIV infection (seropositivity) in conjunction with two or more serious opportunistic infections or cancers. This was initially useful for epidemiologists and clinicians in staging and classifying the disease. However, we now know that AIDS represents the final and most severe symptoms of HIV infection, and it is not really distinct from other manifestations of HIV disease. Recently, a new AIDS definition has been developed: evidence of HIV infection (seropositivity) and T_{helper} counts below 200 per cubic millimeter. In adults, frank AIDS almost never occurs before two years of infection.

Early Immune Failure

Previously, the term *ARC* was sometimes used to describe the relatively minor infections or the lesser manifestations of immune system failure. Following are some of the more common opportunistic infections that occur during this time.

Candida   Candida is a species of fungus, similar to baker's yeast, that can be found on the skin and mucosal surfaces (mouth, vagina) of most people. Normally, Candida growth is held in check by an ecological balance with other microorganisms and by the immune system. With AIDS patients, Candida will often infect the mouth, causing a condition known as *candidiasis* or *thrush*. With thrush, the Candida will form in the mouth white plaques that feel furry to the patient (Figure 5–2). Anti-fungal drugs such as mycostatin are used to control these infections, although they are difficult to completely eliminate.

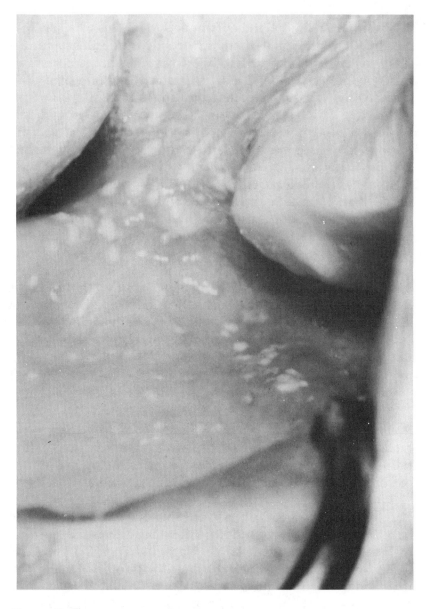

Figure 5–2

Oral Candidiasis. The photograph shows the inside of the mouth, with the gums, cheek, and tongue (on the right). The white spots are areas of *Candida* (yeast) infection.

HIV-infected people who develop candidiasis have a high probability of progressing to frank AIDS. Often, the infection can spread down the esophagus and cause a very painful burning sensation when the patient eats. This condition is known as *esophagitis*; patients with esophagitis are generally considered to have frank AIDS. Approximately 50 percent of AIDS patients will experience, at some time, a Candida infection.

Shingles (varicella)   *Shingles* or *varicella* is a painful rash condition that often occurs on the torso (Figure 5–3). It is caused by the reactivation of a latent virus called *Varicella zoster*. This is the virus that causes chicken pox during childhood; it is a member of the Herpes virus family. After the initial childhood infection, the virus can remain dormant in the nerve trunks for many years and become reactivated when the immune system is compromised or stressed. With AIDS patients, the severity of shingles appears to be greater than that seen in non-AIDS patients, presumably due to their failing immune systems. The antiviral drug acyclovir is sometimes used to help control shingles.

Hairy leukoplakia   This is an abnormal condition of the mouth in which white plaques appear on the surfaces of the tongue. These plaques are not due to the overgrowth of a fungus or bacteria, however. They are due to the abnormal growth of the papillae cells of the tongue; these plaques cannot be scrapped off. These overgrown cells resemble cancer cells and appear to result from infection with another virus called *Epstein-Barr virus*. Epstein-Barr virus is also a member of the Herpes virus family and is the virus that causes infectious mononucleosis in young adults. Hairy leukoplakia is a condition unique to AIDS patients.

Frank AIDS

As discussed elsewhere in this book (Chapters 4 and 6), most HIV-infected individuals will develop some of the symptoms associated with AIDS within eight to ten years after initial infection. The rate at which infected individuals develop symptoms may vary somewhat among different risk groups. For instance,

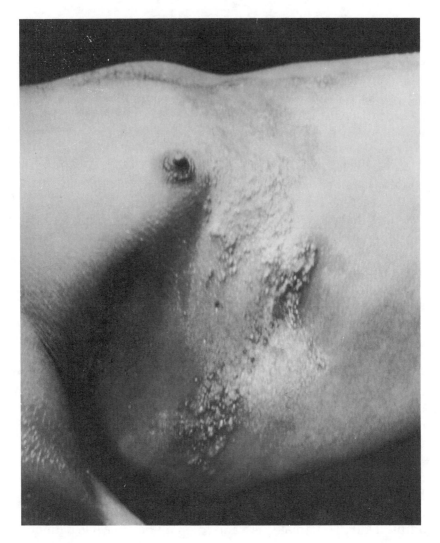

Figure 5–3

Shingles. Reactivation of the latent *varicella Zoster* (chicken pox virus) infection is shown in a band across the torso.

hemophiliacs who were infected by transfusions or blood products may develop AIDS at a slower rate than do gay men. This may be influenced by the number and nature of other microorganisms (potentially opportunistic infections) that these people encounter. The following infections and cancers seen in AIDS patients are indications that the immune system has undergone a catastrophic failure and can no longer prevent life-threatening infections or cancers.

Fungal Infections

Pneumocystis **pneumonia (PCP)**   This illness, which results from inflammation of the lungs, is by far the most common of the serious secondary infections seen with AIDS. About half of all AIDS patients will eventually develop pneumocystis pneumonia, and it is the leading cause of death in AIDS patients. Inflamed areas of the lungs make them appear as white spots in lung X rays (Figure 5–4). The inflammation is caused by infection with fungus called *Pneumocystis carinii*. (Until recently, this microorganism was often classified as a protozoan, but it is now considered a fungus, based on molecular biological studies.) This microorganism gets its name from the person who discovered it, Carini, and from the fact that it can grow into cysts in the lungs of rats (pneumocystis). *Pneumocystis carinii* is relatively common, and small numbers of the fungus can be found in the lungs of healthy people as well as in many animals. It will cause disease in these animals if their immune systems are suppressed. In AIDS patients, the infection is often insidious, and the patient may be unaware of the seriousness of his or her illness. A dry cough is common, and a progressive shortness of breath indicates poor lung function. The shortness of breath is due to the inability of the inflamed lungs to take up adequate amounts of oxygen, which can lead to tissue damage throughout the body. *Pneumocystis carinii* particles are detected by staining the fluid washed out of the lungs with a special dye. PCP can be treated with various antibiotics called *sulfa drugs*. The anti-parasitic agents trimethoprim and sulfamethoxazole (TMP-SMX) are usually given together to control the infection. Another drug called *pentamidine* is also used, especially when TMP-SMX becomes

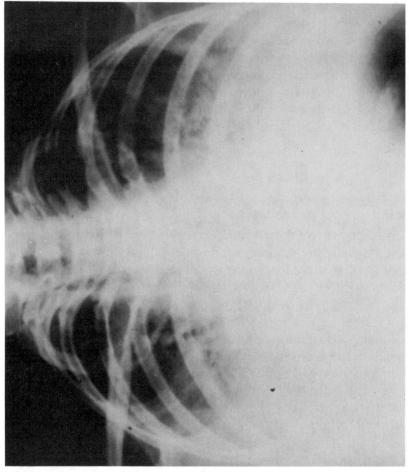

(a)

Figure 5–4

Pneumocystis carinii pneumonia. (a) A chest X ray of an individual with PCP is shown. The ribs are apparent in the top of the X ray, but they are not clear in the bottom. This is because the lungs inside the rib cage are filled with fluid, and they make that area of the X ray appear lighter. In a normal individual, the ribs would be evident against a clear background at the bottom of the picture as well. (*Courtesy of the Centers for Disease Control*); (b) *Opposite*. Lung tissue from an individual with PCP is shown under the light microscope after having been stained. The dark round particles are *pneumocystis* microorganisms within the lung tissue (gray areas).

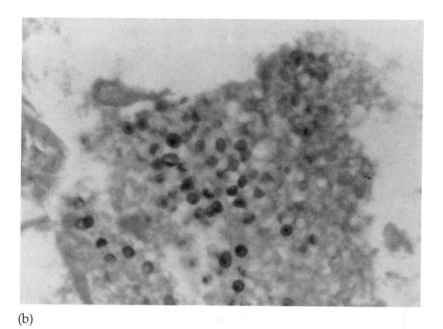

(b)

toxic to the patient. Although these antibiotic treatments are of-ten successful, the lung infection can recur. Some drugs (Fancidar) may be given to prevent recurrences. New drugs, such as trimethexate (an anticancer drug) may also be effective against PCP.

Systemic mycosis   There are three types of common soil fungi that can cause generalized infections in AIDS patients. These fungi can exist in either a moldlike or a yeastlike form and are called *dimorphic*. The three types are *histoplasmosis, coccidio-mycosis*, and *cryptococcus*. These fungi can cause lung infections in healthy people, but generalized or systemic infections are very rare. In AIDS patients, these fungi can cause devastating sys-temic infections that are massive and very widespread. The brain, skin, bone, liver, and lymphatic tissue may all be highly infected. This will typically lead to death of the patient. Antifun-gal drugs such as miconazole are used to control these infections.

Protozoal Infections

***Cryptosporidium* gastroenteritis**   This disease is caused by a protozoan called *cryptosporidium*. This protozoan infects the linings of the intestinal tract and causes diarrhea (gastroenteritis). In healthy people, diarrhea from a cryptosporidium infection is normally mild, lasting only a few days. However, in AIDS patients, the diarrhea is prolonged and severe. The AIDS patient may have from 20 to 50 watery stools per day, accompanied by abdominal cramps and profound weight loss. As a result, there is a serious loss of fluid and electrolytes (salts in the blood). For treatment, patients are given fluids and electrolytes intravenously, and their diarrhea can be controlled somewhat with drugs that slow down intestinal action. However, there is currently no standard antibiotic recognized for use against cryptosporidium. Spiramycin, which is currently an experimental drug, may help to control this persistent infection, but it does not eradicate it. Only about 5 percent of AIDS patients develop this disease. Cryptosporidium also infects cattle and other animals, especially their young; these animals may be the source of human infection.

Toxoplasmosis   This disease is caused by species of protozoa called *Toxoplasma gondii*, which normally causes an asymptomatic infection in healthy adults. This protozoan also infects a very wide variety of animals; domestic cats are one source of human infection. Unlike cryptosporidium, toxoplasma is an intracellular parasite and can invade numerous organs of infected individuals. In AIDS patients, the brain is often infected, which may result in symptoms similar to those seen with brain tumors: convulsions, disorientation, and dementia (Figure 5–5). A CT (computed tomography) scan is used to diagnose toxoplasmosis. For treatment, various antibiotics such as pyrimethamine and sulfadiazine are effective, but they must be administered indefinitely to prevent a relapse. Unfortunately, some patients develop toxic reactions to these drugs.

Bacterial Infections

Interestingly, infections by commonly occurring bacteria (such as those in the lower intestines) do not generally occur in adult AIDS patients, perhaps due to the fact that components of

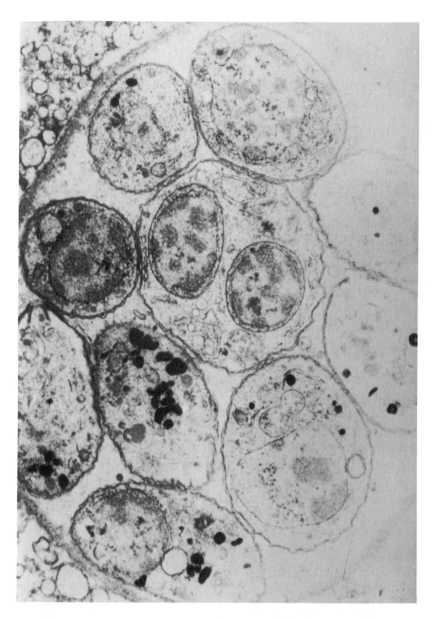

Figure 5–5

Toxoplasmosis. An electron microscope picture of a *toxoplasma* cyst is shown. A cyst is a walled-off area of microorganisms within a tissue. Each of the round areas in the photograph is a cross-section of a *toxoplasma* microorganism. (*Courtesy of the Centers for Disease Control*) the immune system responsible for controlling the common bacteria are less affected by HIV infection. However, children born infected with AIDS often do develop lung infections with common bacteria. In addition, adult AIDS patients may experience infections with tuberculosis-like bacteria.

Mycobacterium   This is a genus of bacteria that has characteristic cell walls with unusual staining properties in the laboratory. The bacterium that causes tuberculosis is a member of this genus. AIDS patients are most commonly infected with an atypical form of tuberculosis bacterium called *Mycobacterium avium-intrecellulare*. This bacterium does not normally cause disease in healthy people, but in AIDS patients, it may cause a tuberculosis-like disease in the lungs. The infection can also involve numerous other tissues, such as the bone marrow, and bacteria may be present in the blood at very high levels (Figure 5–6). Patients with this opportunistic infection will have fevers and low numbers of white blood cells. These infections are often resistant to drugs and are often treated with the simultaneous administration of up to six different antibiotics. Isoniazid and rifampin are usually among the drugs used. This type of infection is more common in AIDS patients who were IV drug users.

More recently, standard tuberculosis has become a common infection in AIDS patients. TB was largely eradicated in the United States by the mid-1970s through public health measures and antibiotic treatments. However, recently there has been a resurgence of TB, due to a combination of several factors: (1) increased immigration from areas where TB infection is still common (developing countries in Asia and Latin America); (2) a decline in funding for public health care measures, which has allowed TB to spread; and (3) AIDS patients, who are highly susceptible to TB infection and who in turn can transmit the bacterium. A very disturbing trend is the increasing appearance of TB strains that are resistant to antibiotics. This probably results from incomplete therapy of TB patients: In order to eradicate the bacteria from these individuals, a lengthy course of antibiotics is required, with repeated follow-up and testing until the bacteria are completely eliminated. However, if follow-up is incomplete, even if most of the TB bacteria are eliminated, the surviving bac-

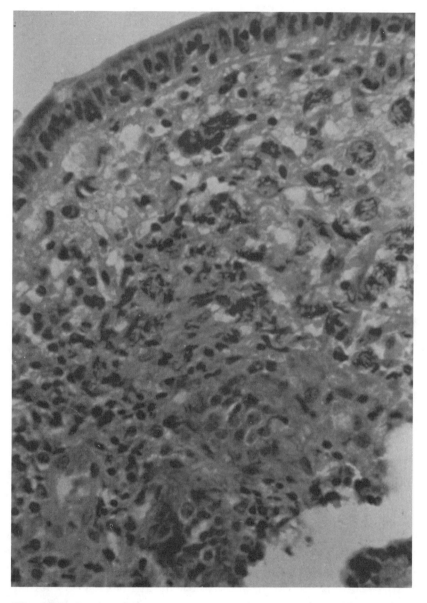

Figure 5–6

Mycobacterium. A section of the small bowel is shown under the light microscope. The dark particles in the center of the photograph represent *Mycobacterium avium-intracellularae* particles within the bowel tissue. (*Courtesy of the Centers for Disease Control*) teria can reestablish and spread to other individuals once antibiotic therapy is stopped. In addition, these bacteria will frequently be resistant to the antibiotic that was administered. Tuberculosis is now a major threat to health-care workers, particularly in hospital settings where there are large numbers of indigent individuals, including AIDS patients.

Viral Infections

Cytomegalovirus   This is a member of the Herpes virus family, as are the varicella zoster and Epstein-Barr viruses described earlier. Cytomegalovirus (CMV) is a common virus, and many people are infected early in childhood. Children tend to get an asymptomatic infection, while infected young adults may develop a mononucleosis-like illness. Infection of a fetus (a congenital infection) is very serious and can lead to permanent brain damage or death of the fetus. In AIDS patients, CMV infection can recur and tends to infect the retinas of eyes, leading to blindness. The virus also infects the adrenal gland, leading to hormonal imbalance. Pneumonia, fever, rash, and gastroenteritis due to CMV infection are also seen in AIDS patients. CMV pneumonia in patients who have PCP at the same time is usually fatal. The antiviral drug gancyclovir (related to acyclovir; see above) may help control CMV infections.

Cancers

Kaposi's sarcoma   These are tumors of the blood vessels (Figure 5–7). In non-AIDS patients, Kaposi's sarcoma (KS) is typically only seen in older men of Mediterranean or Jewish ancestry. In homosexual men with AIDS, up to 69 percent may develop Kaposi's sarcoma. Initially, only a few tumors appear as pink, purple, or brown skin lesions, usually located on the arms or legs. These tumors will spread and become widely distributed, eventually involving most of the linings of the body. If they spread to the lungs, they are difficult to control. Chemotherapy can now eradicate these tumors with a high success rate. Triaziquone, actinomycin D, bleomycin, and ICRF-159 are often used in chemotherapy. AIDS patients with KS often have a high level of opportunistic infections.

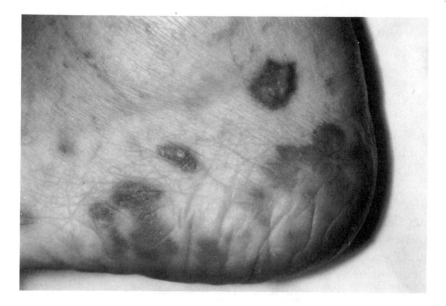

Figure 5–7

Kaposi's sarcoma. Dark (purplish) areas of Kaposi's sarcoma are shown on the heel of the foot.

Lymphomas   The lymphomas that occur in AIDS patients are cancers derived from the B-cells of the immune system. These are cells that make antibodies, as discussed in Chapter 3. Reactivation or co-infection in the B-lymphocytes with Epstein-Barr virus may be important for development of the lymphomas. As mentioned previously in this chapter, the Epstein-Barr virus causes mononucleosis in young adults, but it can also transform normal B-cells into cancer cells. In AIDS patients, an unusual lymphoma that spreads to the brain also occurs.

Cervical Cancer   In female AIDS patients, cancer of the cervix (a part of the female genital tract) is also observed at high frequency. Cervical cancer is a fairly common cancer in women, although it typically affects women of middle age or older. Infection with certain strains of human papilloma virus (HPV) that cause warts in the genital tract is an underlying cause of cervical cancer. Like HIV, genital infection of HPV occurs by sexual contact. Thus, in AIDS patients, this HPV virus-induced cancer develops more rapidly in the absence of a normal immune system.

This list of opportunistic infections and cancers seen in AIDS patients only covers the most commonly observed diseases. Numerous other infections are also seen at lower frequencies. In addition, an individual patient may experience a combination of these illnesses. It is interesting that there are characteristic cancers and opportunistic infection in AIDS patients. These diseases are only a fraction of potential diseases that could affect an immunocompromised person. This may be due to the fact that HIV more seriously damages certain parts of the immune system. In addition, other factors, such as previously established chronic or latent infections, may be important. Once the immune system fails, these preexisting infections can then proliferate and cause disease symptoms.

AZT TREATMENT IN AIDS

In order to restore the health of an AIDS patient, it will be necessary to suppress the replication of HIV and to rebuild the damaged immune system (see Chapter 11). So far, this is beyond our technical capacity. Certainly, antiviral drugs will play an important role in the clinical treatment of this disease. Currently, azidothymidine (AZT) is the primary drug used in alleviating AIDS (see Chapters 4 and 6). AIDS patients who are given AZT show increased survival. Without AZT, the average life expectancy of an AIDS patient who has an opportunistic infection is about six months. With AZT, that life expectancy rises to one-and-a-half years. Treatment with AZT actually results in some recovery of immune function. The number of T_{helper} lymphocytes in AZT-treated AIDS patients increases; they experience fewer opportunistic infections, and they may actually gain weight. The patients also feel better.

For other viral illnesses, the infections have never yet been completely eradicated with an antiviral drug. However, with AIDS it may only be necessary to prevent high levels of virus replication in order to control the disease.

The cost of AZT is high—about $3,500 per year for one person. Current treatment regimens demand that a patient take an AZT pill once every four hours, around the clock. As mentioned in Chapter 4, AZT treatment has some side effects, such as nausea, headache, and loss of sleep. The major complication is that about half of treated patients will become anemic and have a low white blood cell count. This in itself can lead to an increase in bacterial infections. If anemia occurs, AZT treatment must be discontinued, at least temporarily.

Earlier preliminary studies indicate that AZT treatment is also effective in asymptomatic HIV-infected individuals. That is, AZT treatment of these people slowed the rate at which their immune systems declined. Moreover, some of the toxic side effects (anemia) occurred less frequently in these individuals. This led to the general recommendation that individuals who suspect that they may have been exposed to HIV have themselves tested (under conditions that ensure counseling and confidentiality). Their immune systems can then be monitored (e.g., T_{helper} lymphocyte counts; see chapter 4) for signs of damage, and opportunistic infections can be monitored as well. Preventive therapies such as AZT and aerosol pentamidine (to prevent PCP) can then be used before the individual becomes seriously ill. Seriously ill patients are much more difficult to treat medically.

Very recently, the effectiveness of AZT in treatment of HIV and AIDS has been called into question by a large clinical trial held in England and France , the Concorde trial. In this study, asymptomatic HIV-infected individuals were treated with AZT and compared with a matched group who received no drug. The study found that there was no difference in the rate of AIDS-related deaths between the AZT-treated and untreated individuals. Thus, the advisability of treating asymptomatic HIV-infected people with AZT is now uncertain. However, it is possible that the relatively high doses of AZT used in the Concorde trial may have been a negative factor in the health of the AZT-treated people. Other preliminary results suggest that lower doses of AZT in healthy asymptomatic HIV-infected individuals may have a beneficial effect. At the same time, AZT clearly has a positive effect in extending and improving the quality of life in AIDS patients (see Table 6–5)—that is, if it is administered for the first time to individuals once they have developed symptoms. Currently, there is considerable discussion among doctors about the best way to use AZT to combat HIV infection and AIDS.

Recently, two additional antiviral drugs have been approved for treatment of AIDS: dideoxyinosine (DDI) and dideoxycytidine (DDC). Like AZT, both DDI and DDC are anologues of DNA building blocks that terminate further DNA synthesis if incorporated into DNA by HIV reverse transcriptase more efficiently than by cellular DNA polymerases. DDI has been approved as an alternative drug for HIV-infected individuals who cannot tolerate AZT. DDC has been approved for use in combination with AZT. One of the theoretical advantages for combination treatment with AZT and DDC or DDI is that HIV variants that become resistant to AZT may still be sensitive to DDC or DDI. Like AZT, both DDI and DDC cause side effects in some patients. Some individuals taking DDI develop pancreatitis (a serious inflammation of the pancreas), and some individuals on DDC experience peripheral neuropathies (tingling in the extremities).

Chapter 6
Epidemiology and AIDS

In the preceding chapter, we considered how HIV manifests itself in an infected individual. The next level of complexity will be to consider how HIV moves between individuals and its effects on populations. For these topics, the discipline of epidemiology is very important. The modes of HIV transmission and relative risk factors are addressed in the following chapter. This chapter gives an overview of epidemiology, with some applications regarding HIV and AIDS.

Epidemiology is the study of the patterns of disease occurrence in populations and of the factors affecting them. This field is of great importance to the understanding of human diseases, and epidemiological studies can be used to address many questions.

What can epidemiology tell us about diseases? Epidemiological studies can:

- *Identify new diseases.*
- *Identify populations at risk for a disease.*
- *Identify possible causative agents of a disease.*
- *Identify factors or behaviors that increase risk of a disease.*

They can also determine the relative importance of a factor in contributing to a disease.

- *Rule out factors or behaviors as contributing to a disease.*
- *Evaluate therapies for a disease.*
- *Guide the development of effective public health measures and preventative strategies.*

It is important to keep in mind that epidemiological studies involve large groups or *populations* of individuals. This approach gives great power to these studies since they draw on the total experience and behavior of large numbers of individuals.

The fact that epidemiological studies are based on observation of groups also introduces some limitations and risks in interpretations. One limitation is that these studies cannot predict how any individual person will be affected by a factor even if the population as a whole is affected by that factor. Epidemiological studies also cannot predict the course a disease will take in a particular person. Some risks are associated with drawing improper conclusions from epidemiology. For instance, it is important to avoid making an ecological fallacy—explaining behavior of an individual based on observations of an entire group. Another example of improper conclusions is identifying certain characteristics of a group as causing a disease. For example, epidemiological studies have identified male homosexuals as one of the groups at high risk for AIDS. This does not imply that simply being homosexual causes AIDS, as some people have claimed. Instead, certain sexual behaviors by some gay men link them to AIDS, as we shall see later in this chapter and also in Chapter 7.

Despite these limitations and risks, epidemiological studies provide some of the most definitive information about the causes and dynamics of human diseases, short of carrying out experiments on humans.

AN OVERVIEW OF EPIDEMIOLOGY AND AIDS

Epidemiology has played a central role in the fight against AIDS right from the beginning, and this will continue. The initial identification of AIDS as a new syndrome in 1981 was made by epidemiological studies. These studies reported the unusually high occurrence of individuals with rare diseases associated with immunological defects (see Chapter 1). The initial epidemiological studies showed a high frequency of the new disease in sexually active male homosexuals. Furthermore, the pattern of occurrences suggested that AIDS might be caused by an infectious agent, which could be transmitted by sexual means. Subsequently, the appearance of AIDS cases among recipients of blood transfusions or blood products (for instance, hemophiliacs) as well as intravenous drug abusers suggested that AIDS could be transmitted through contaminated blood. The study of individuals afflicted with AIDS and also of groups of high-risk individuals led to the isolation in 1984 of HIV, the virus that causes AIDS. As soon as HIV was isolated, the virus was used to develop the test for HIV antibodies (see Chapter 4). The availability of the HIV antibody test allowed much more accurate epidemiological studies since evidence of infection could also be detected in healthy asymptomatic individuals. This led to the realization that an alarming number of individuals have been infected with HIV in many parts of the world. Moreover, we are currently only seeing the tip of the HIV iceberg, since it often takes several years for the disease to develop. Epidemiological studies of high-risk groups have identified the underlying high-risk behaviors, such as unprotected sexual intercourse and sharing IV needles. This, in turn, has led to development of public health measures and safe-sex guidelines, which are our only weapons in AIDS prevention today. Finally, epidemiological studies (which also could be classified as clinical studies) provided the proof that azidothymidine (AZT) is an effective therapeutic drug for AIDS.

BASIC CONCEPTS IN EPIDEMIOLOGY

There are two basic kinds of epidemiological studies: *descriptive* and *analytical*. The goal of the first is to describe the occurrence of disease in populations. Analytical studies seek to identify and explain the causes of diseases. Frequently, descriptive epidemiological studies will lead to analytical studies. For instance, descriptive epidemiology may identify a new disease, such as AIDS, or suggest hypotheses about the causes of a disease. Interpretation of the descriptive studies will then suggest hypotheses leading to analytical studies that examine the disease in more detail.

Since epidemiology is the study of disease in populations, the proportion of affected individuals in a population is of basic importance. There are two important measures used in epidemiology:

> *Prevalence.* This is the fraction (or proportion) of current living individuals in a population who have a disease or infection at a particular time.

Incidence. This is the proportion of a population that develops *new* cases of a disease or infection during a particular time period.

As an example, let's look at Table 6–1. It shows the number of individuals with evidence of previous infection with hepatitis virus (antibodies for the virus) in a city for the years 1968 and 1988. During this time, the size of the city has also increased from 100,000 to 150,000. The *prevalence* of hepatitis virus infection was 0.5 percent in 1968, and it increased to 0.67 percent in 1988. The *incidence* of infection during this period was 0.17 percent (0.67 percent minus 0.5 percent); put another way, this means that per 100,000 people, there were 170 new cases of infection during the 20-year period. The *yearly* incidence rate would be 0.17 percent divided by 20 (0.0085 percent new cases per 100,000 people per year). Epidemiologists use these prevalence and incidence data to calculate other expressions of their results, such as risk values.

DESCRIPTIVE STUDIES

Descriptive epidemiological studies measure the appearance of disease by categories of *person, place,* and *time.* An example of disease appearance by person is the observation that lung cancer predominantly appears in individuals who smoke cigarettes

Table 6–1
HEPATITIS VIRUS INFECTION IN A CITY*

	1968	**1988**
Total population	100,000	150,000
Individuals with hepatitis virus antibodies (seropositives)	500	1,000
Prevalence of seropositive individuals	0.5% (500/100,000)	0.67% (1,000/150,000)

*This is an example for discussion only. There are actually three different viruses that can cause hepatitis.

(*person* = smokers). Disease appearance by place would be studies showing the low incidence of tooth decay in areas where there is a high level of naturally occurring fluorides in the water supply (*place* = high-fluoride areas). Disease appearance by time would be an outbreak of food poisoning resulting from contaminated food at a picnic (*time* = days after the picnic).

An important concept in descriptive epidemiology is clustering. *Clustering* is the unusually high incidence *or* prevalence of a disease in a subpopulation. Clustering can occur by person, place, or time, or a combination of them. The first documented outbreak of Legionnaire's disease is a good example of clustering. Legionnaire's disease is a serious bacterial respiratory infection that can be fatal if untreated. The disease was first identified among several members of the American Legion who attended an American Legion convention at a hotel in Philadelphia in the summer of 1976. Thus, the disease was clustered with respect to place (the hotel in Philadelphia), time (1976), and person (American Legion members). Ultimately, a new microorganism (*Legionella*) was isolated, which causes Legionnaire's disease.

Types of Descriptive Epidemiological Studies

Descriptive epidemiological studies are carried out according to several design strategies or a combination of these strategies. Two of the important strategies are *case reports* or *case report series* and *cross-sectional* or *prevalence studies*.

Case reports/case report series   Case reports are descriptions of an unusual disease occurrence in individual patients. Sometimes the nature of the case may also suggest a relationship between some predisposing factor and the disease or it may suggest the appearance of a new disease. These suggestions are strengthened if several similar cases are observed and reported together—a *case report series*. The original report in 1981 by Gottlieb describing pneumocystis pneumonia in six homosexual men is a classic example of a case report series (see Chapter 1). This report suggested that a new disease (AIDS) might be occurring and that male homosexuals were at high risk.

Cross-sectional/prevalence studies   In these studies, a population is monitored for the occurrence of a disease or a series of diseases, and statistics about each case (nature of the patient, geographical location) are recorded. This information can be used to construct a cross-sectional profile for the disease or diseases within the population. These studies are also sometimes carried out over a long period of time, and the date of disease occurrence is also recorded. Once the cross-sectional profile is obtained, then it can be examined for clustering of disease cases by person, place, or time. These clusterings can suggest causes of known diseases and also identify new ones.

Cancer registries are an example of these studies. In these registries, information is gathered on all cases of cancer occurring in a region. Information from the cancer registry can then be used by cancer epidemiologists to investigate potential causes of cancer. For instance, these registries have provided strong evidence for a causal relationship between cigarette smoking and lung cancer.

The United States Public Health Service maintains a registry of deaths and diseases, which is reported on a weekly basis in a journal called the *Morbidity and Mortality Weekly Report*. Information from this registry was also important in characterizing the AIDS epidemic in 1981 and 1982, since there was a sharp increase in cases of pneumocystis pneumonia and Kaposi's sarcoma at that time. The U.S. Public Health Service now publishes a monthly HIV/AIDS surveillance report that provides current and past epidemiological information exclusively on HIV infection and AIDS.

Prevalence studies can also be used to identify groups within the population that are at higher risk for a particular disease. Besides suggesting possible causes of the disease, this information can be used for other purposes as well. First, if the disease is rare in the overall population, it will be more efficient to study the disease by focusing on the high-risk population—this is important for analytical epidemiology (see below). Second, public health workers may want to focus particular attention on the high-risk population as a first step in working out prevention strategies to combat the disease.

ANALYTICAL STUDIES

Analytical epidemiology studies are generally more focused than descriptive studies. They investigate the causes of a particular disease, and they often involve assigning a numerical value to (quantifying) a potential risk factor. In fact, the distinction between descriptive and analytical studies is not absolute. Most epidemiological studies fall somewhere between a completely descriptive study and a purely analytical one. For instance, cancer registries can be used for analytical epidemiology studies, in which the relationship between a particular factor and a disease (for instance, smoking and lung cancer) is examined in detail, and the relative risk is determined.

Types of Analytical Epidemiological Studies

There are two main approaches to analytical epidemiology: *experimental* or *interventional studies* and *observational studies*.

Experimental/interventional studies   In these studies, a condition of an experimental subpopulation is changed, and the effect on the development of a disease is observed. The results are compared with the main population or an untreated subpopulation. This approach has been very useful in testing potential therapies for diseases. For instance, the Salk polio vaccine was tested in a nationwide trial of second- and third-grade school children in 1953–1954. The success of the trial led to the acceptance of the vaccine and the elimination of polio as a major health threat. A more recent example is a test of a vaccine for Hepatitis B virus. This vaccine was tested in a population of sexually active male homosexuals (who are also at high risk for Hepatitis B infection) and shown to be very effective. Clinical drug trials can also be considered interventional epidemiology.

While interventional studies are very useful in testing therapies, it is often difficult to use them to directly test if a factor causes a disease. Treating a group of people with a factor that might cause a disease raises serious ethical questions. This is particularly important if, as is the case for AIDS, there is no effective cure for the disease. One possible solution to this dilemma is to see if the same disease can be induced by the factor in animals. Another approach is that of observational epidemiology.

Observational studies   Observational studies take advantage of the fact that within a population, certain individuals will encounter a factor and develop a disease while others will not. The epidemiologist does not change the conditions of people to study the disease but rather *subdivides* the population according to possible risk factors or disease and studies them separately. For instance, by subdividing a population into cigarette smokers and nonsmokers, the epidemiologist can investigate the effect of cigarette smoking on cancer or heart disease without making anybody smoke. In some cases, a properly designed observational study can provide the same information as an interventional study.

There are two main types of observational studies: *case/control studies* and *cohort* studies.

Case/control studies involve studying a group of individuals with a particular disease (the cases) and comparing them with a group of unaffected individuals (the controls). The controls are often matched for a number of factors not believed to be involved in the disease. If the cases differ from the controls by another factor as well, this would suggest that the factor is related to the disease. For instance, if lung cancer patients are compared to individuals without lung cancer, a higher percentage of the cancer patients are cigarette smokers than in the control population.

Case/control studies are particularly useful if the disease being studied only occurs rarely. For instance, if a disease only occurs once per million people in the United States, it would be impractical to survey everybody in the population to study those few cases that occur. On the other hand, nationally, there would be about 200 cases of the disease, which could be readily studied by the case/control approach. For the same reason, case/control studies are important at the beginning of infectious disease epidemics, when there are still very few cases. The early epidemiology studies in the AIDS epidemic were mainly case/control studies.

Cohort studies focus on a group of individuals who share a particular risk factor for a disease. This group is then examined for the frequency or rate of disease appearance in comparison to a control population that does not have the risk factor. Such studies can implicate or exonerate a potential risk factor for the disease, and they can also determine the degree to which the risk factor contributes to the disease.

Cohort studies can go forward or backward in time. *Prospective* cohort studies go forward in time, starting with an identified cohort of individuals and documenting development of disease as time progresses. A number of cohort studies for AIDS are presently underway, principally involving gay or bisexual men. For instance, one cohort study involves HIV antibody-positive individuals, and the occurrence of lymphadenopathy syndrome (LAS), ARC, and AIDS is being tracked. In another study, a group of single men in San Francisco are being followed for infection with HIV, and the factors (sexual practices, IV drug use) associated with infection are being studied.

Cohort studies that go back in time are called *retrospective* studies. In these studies, exposure to the risk factor has occurred previously, and the cohort of individuals is later identified for observation. For instance, retrospective cohort studies have been carried out on individuals who worked in asbestos-processing plants in the 1940s and 1950s. These individuals subsequently showed a high incidence of lung cancer, implicating asbestos as another potential cause of lung cancer.

Correlations

In analytical epidemiology, results are considered in terms of *statistical associations* or *correlations* between a factor and a disease. For instance, a high frequency of cigarette smoking is found among lung cancer patients, which means there is a statistical association between cigarette smoking and lung cancer. The aim of analytical epidemiology is to deduce *causality* from the statistical association—in our example, that cigarette smoking causes lung cancer. However, there are other possible explanations for statistical associations.

There are three possible reasons for a positive correlation between a factor and a disease:

1. There is no causal relationship. This could result from faulty design of the experiment. For instance, if the control population is not properly matched with the experimental population, a false correlation could be observed.

2. There is an *indirect* relationship. In some situations there may be a third *confounding* variable that influences both the factor being tested and the disease. For instance, there is a positive statistical correlation between alcohol consumption and lung cancer, but this does not mean that alcohol causes lung cancer. In this case, cigarette smoking is a confounding variable. Cigarette smoking causes lung cancer, *and* cigarette smoking is also statistically associated with alcohol consumption. That is, individuals who are cigarette smokers also tend to drink more alcohol than do nonsmokers.

   Another example of an indirect relationship is the high statistical correlation between swim suit sales and ice cream sales. This does not mean that ice cream consumption leads to swim suit purchases, or vice versa. In this case, summer or high temperature is a confounding variable. More swim suits are bought during the summer, when it is warm and beach weather is good, and more people eat ice cream during this time because it is hot.

3. There is a *direct* causal relationship. That is, a change in the factor will lead to a change in occurrence of the disease. However, it is important to remember that more than one factor can be a direct cause of a disease. Thus, establishment of a direct causal relationship between one factor and a disease does not rule out other factors as well.

Criteria for a Causal Relationship

In observational studies, it is difficult to absolutely prove a causal relationship from a correlation because the epidemiologist does not change the factors under study. However, there are criteria that provide tests for causality. These criteria are:

1. *Strength of the association* between the factor and the disease. The strongest correlation would be if everybody with the factor gets the disease, and nobody without the factor gets the disease. A strong correlation makes a causal relationship more likely. The argument is also strengthened if there is a dose-response relationship—that is, if individuals who have received higher exposure to a factor show higher frequencies of disease. However, it is always important to keep in mind that confounding variables could exist.
2. *Consistency* of the association. That is, if the same correlation is observed in other studies, using different settings and different populations.
3. The association has the *correct time relationship*. That is, exposure to the agent must occur *before* development of the disease.
4. The association has *biological plausibility*. That is, association of the factor with the disease makes biological sense.

For infectious agents, another set of rules has been developed for assessing if a microbe causes a disease: *Koch's postulates*. Koch's postulates are discussed in Chapter 2, and they require both observational and experimental studies. Briefly, a microorganism can be considered the cause of a disease if (1) it is always found in diseased individuals, (2) it can be isolated from the diseased individual and grown pure in culture, (3) the pure microorganism can cause the disease when introduced into susceptible individuals, and (4) the same microorganism can be reisolated from those individuals.

EPIDEMIOLOGY AND AIDS IN THE UNITED STATES

Let us now see what epidemiology can tell us about AIDS in more detail. As described in the overview in this chapter, epidemiology has been extremely important in this epidemic. Let's look at some of the epidemiological information and the conclusions that can be drawn from it.

The Current Picture of AIDS in the United States

Figure 6–1 shows the total number of AIDS cases that have been reported in the United States for the years 1981 through 1991. By October 1992, a total of 240,000 cases had been reported, of which 160,000 had died. Current estimates are that between 800,000 and 1 million people in the United States are currently infected with HIV; a sizable fraction of these people are likely to develop AIDS and ultimately to die if new therapies are not found. Thus, we can see the seriousness of this epidemic and the strain that it will place on our society.

Figure 6–2 shows the distribution of AIDS cases according to risk groups. Homosexual and bisexual men make up the largest percentage of cases, followed by injection drug users, hemophiliacs and recipients of blood transfusions, sexual partners of HIV-infected individuals, and children of HIV-infected mothers. For a small percentage of cases (about 4 percent), no risk group has been assigned. However, many of these may be due to the unavailability of information about the patients or the reluctance of patients to acknowledge membership in a high-risk group. Women make up 11 percent of American AIDS cases; this low percentage is due to the fact that the largest number of cases occur in homosexual and bisexual men. Women make up about half of the AIDS cases for the other risk groups.

The distribution of AIDS cases shown in Figure 6–2 represents the cumulative totals from the beginning of the epidemic. The distribution among different risk groups may change with time. For instance, most of the AIDS cases associated with blood transfusions or blood products resulted from HIV infections before 1985. At that time, the HIV antibody test became available to protect the nation's blood supply. Now that the risk of infection from blood transfusions has been greatly reduced, the percentage of new AIDS cases resulting from transfusions will decrease in the future. Also, behavior modifications that decrease high-risk behaviors will change these percentages. In San Francisco, a concerted educational campaign targeted at the gay male community has markedly reduced the rate of new HIV infections in that high-risk group. On the other hand, if HIV infection spreads further within high-risk groups or into other populations, then

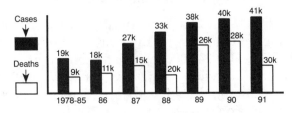

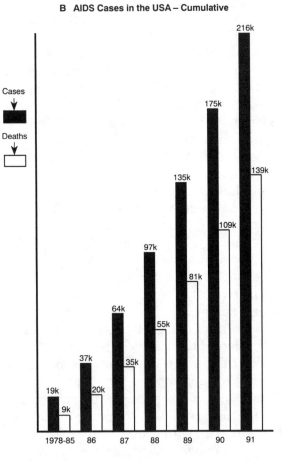

Figure 6–1

Appearance of AIDS in the USA. Data compiled from the September 1992 HIV/AIDS Surveillance Report from the U.S. Centers for Disease Control.

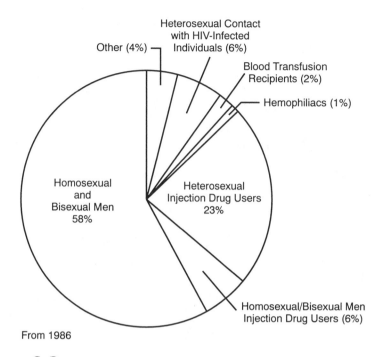

From 1986

Figure 6–2

Distribution of AIDS cases by risk groups. (Cumulative figures, 1981–September, 1992)

cases among these groups will increase. For instance, HIV infection is currently spreading virtually unchecked among injection drug users in the New York metropolitan area. In this area, more than 70 percent of individuals who use injection drugs are HIV infected. Indeed, in this area, injection drug users make up a majority of the *new* AIDS cases. At the present time, other geographical areas have lower rates of HIV infection in the injection drug user population, but if infection spreads in these areas, then a marked shift in distribution of AIDS cases may occur.

Figure 6–3 shows the distribution of AIDS cases according to ethnicity. There is a disproportional number of AIDS cases among minorities, particularly African Americans and Hispanics. Indeed, while these groups make up about 23 percent of the general population, they make up 47 percent of AIDS cases—and an even higher percentage of the cases associated with injection drug use. Put another way, the frequency of AIDS cases among

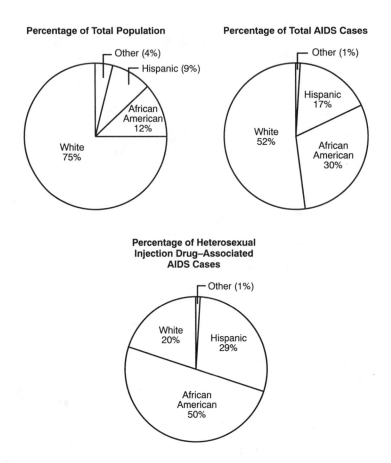

Figure 6–3

AIDS cases by ethnicity. (Cumulative figures, 1981–September, 1992)

African Americans and Hispanics is about twice as high as in the general population. This points out the urgency of developing public health and educational measures targeted to these communities, in order to control the epidemic.

Epidemiology and Modes of HIV Transmission

Transmission of HIV will be addressed in detail in the next chapter. However, some examples of epidemiological studies regarding HIV transmission will be presented here, to illustrate how these studies allow us to draw conclusions about the relative risks of different activities for HIV transmission. One study will implicate an activity (anal sex) in HIV transmission, and another study will show that casual contact does not cause HIV transmission. In addition, the possibility of HIV transmission by insects will be considered.

Anal sex—a high-risk mode   Let's consider a recent epidemiological study that looked at the relative risks of different sexual activities. This study was part of the San Francisco Men's Health Study, which is an ongoing cohort study of single men in an area of San Francisco. This particular area has been particularly hard hit by the AIDS epidemic. The study involves 1,034 single men, who are monitored for HIV antibody status and asked about their sexual practices. Of the homosexual men in this cohort, 48 percent were seropositive at the beginning. A low percentage (17.6 percent) of men who had refrained from sex during the previous two years were seropositive, and this could be traced to sexual activity before that time. Table 6–2 shows frequencies of HIV infection when the homosexual men in the study were divided according to whether or not they practiced

Table 6–2
HIV INFECTION IN HOMOSEXUAL MEN: THE RELATIVE RISK OF ANAL SEX*

Sexual Practices for the Preceding 2 Years	Percent HIV Seropositive (Adjusted for Number of Sexual Contacts)
No anal sex	20.6%
Anal sex, insertive only	26.7%
Anal sex, receptive only	44.6%
Anal sex, both insertive and receptive	53.3%

*These data are from the San Francisco Men's Study, as reported by Winkelstein et al. (J. Amer. Med. Assoc. 257:321 [1987]). Individuals who did not practice anal sex for the previous two years included those who practiced oral sex only and also those who abstained entirely. The strongest correlation for HIV seropositivity in this study was the number of sexual contacts an individual had. The percentages in the table were adjusted to account for the average number of sexual contacts for the different groups.

anal intercourse. Those who were the receptive partner or who were both receptive and insertive showed significantly higher frequencies of HIV infection than those who did not engage in anal sex. This shows that anal intercourse is a high-risk mode of HIV infection.

The results also showed that those who only practiced insertive anal intercourse were at less risk—in fact, this particular study could not statistically distinguish those men from men who did not engage in anal sex at all. However, other studies of heterosexual couples (who engage in vaginal as well as anal intercourse) clearly show that insertive intercourse can result in HIV transmission to the man. Thus, the most likely situation is that anal receptive intercourse is a very high-risk sexual activity, while insertive intercourse is somewhat lower, although significant, in risk.

Casual contact—no measurable risk for HIV transmission *Casual contact* with HIV-infected individuals poses no risk for infection. This was determined early in the epidemic, since people living with AIDS patients did not develop signs of HIV infection or AIDS. Casual contact includes hugging, touching, dry kissing, sharing of eating or drinking utensils, and sharing the workplace, telephones, and the like.

An example of an epidemiological study establishing that casual contact does not lead to HIV infection is shown in Table 6–3. One hundred and one individuals who shared a household with an AIDS patient for at least three months were tested for the presence of HIV antibodies. Only one person was seropositive, and this individual was a child of two injection drug users. Further investigation showed that this child acquired the infection at birth and not through casual contact. Thus, none of the individuals in this study became HIV infected through casual contact.

Insect bites—no evidence for spread of HIV Some people have claimed that insect bites can be a source of infection because insects such as mosquitoes draw a blood meal from a person that they are biting, and they move from person to person. However, epidemiological evidence argues against insect transmission of HIV. First of all, in well-studied North American

Table 6–3

HIV INFECTION IN CASUAL HOUSEHOLD CONTACTS OF AIDS
PATIENTS[1]

	Number Tested	Number HIV Seropositive
Children less than 6 years old	21	1[2]
Offspring of an AIDS patient	15	1[2]
Offspring of others	6	0
Children 6 to 18 years old	47	0
Adults	33	0
Total tested	101	

[1]The subjects in this study had lived in the same household with an AIDS patient for at least three months. Individuals who were in known high-risk groups (sexual relations with the AIDS patient, injection drug use, homosexual men) were not included. Thus, only individuals who had casual contact with the AIDS patient were studied. Among this group, 48 percent shared drinking glasses with the AIDS patient, 25 percent shared eating utensils, 9 percent shared razor blades, 90 percent shared toilets, and 37 percent shared beds. The AIDS patient was hugged by 79 percent of the subjects, kissed on the cheek by 83 percent, and kissed on the lips by 17 percent.

[2]Further investigation showed that the one seropositive child was the offspring of two IV drug abusers, and probably acquired the infection at birth; this is a known mechanism of HIV transmission. Thus, none of these casual household contacts of AIDS patients became infected. These data are taken from a report by Friedland et al. (New England J. Med. 314:3244 [1986]).

or European populations, the great majority (about 97 percent) of AIDS cases can be explained by the well-documented modes of transmission. This includes a recent study in Belle Glade, Florida, where some people proposed an outbreak of AIDS due to insect transmission. Furthermore, in Africa, where the insect populations are high, the age and geographical distributions of HIV infection argue against insect transmission. HIV is rare in children and the elderly, even in households where there are HIV-infected individuals. The old and the young are actually more frequently bitten by mosquitoes and other insects. In terms of geographical distribution, HIV infection is at high frequency in certain cities and urban areas, and there is much lower frequency of infection in surrounding rural areas. This is actually opposite from the pattern that would be expected if insects transmitted HIV, since they are more plentiful in rural areas.

Likelihood of Progression to AIDS

One very important question is the likelihood of an HIV-infected individual eventually developing clinical AIDS. Initial estimates were that perhaps 10 percent of infected individuals would develop the disease. However, more recent studies indicate that a much higher percentage of infected individuals will eventually develop AIDS. Prospective cohort studies have followed HIV-seropositive individuals for development of AIDS or ARC. An example of one study is shown in Table 6–4. After about four years of observation, 18 percent of the seropositive individuals developed AIDS, and an additional 47 percent developed signs of immunological impairment. Only 35 percent remained asymptomatic. Other similar studies currently predict that most individuals infected with HIV (more than 70 percent) will develop AIDS or ARC within eight to ten years of infection.

Table 6–4
LONG-TERM RESULTS OF HIV IN INFECTED MEN*

	Number of Individuals	Percent Total
AIDS	10	17.5
Signs of Immunological Damage		
LAS	16	28.1
Others (oral candidiasis, weight loss, etc.)	11	19.3
Subtotal	27	47.4
Asymptomatic	20	35.1

*Men in this study were followed for an average of 44 months after they showed initial signs of HIV infection (seroconversion). These data are taken from Ward et al. ("AIDS", G.P. Wormser et al., eds., Noyes Publications, Park Ridge, NJ [1987], pp 18–35).

The Effectiveness of AZT

As described in Chapter 3, azidothymidine (AZT) is the only major antiviral agent effective in AIDS. Previous laboratory experiments had shown that the drug could block HIV infection in isolated culture systems, and the drug was tested in a clinical trial, which can also be considered an interventional epidemiological study. Results from the first clinical trial of AZT are shown in Table 6–5. AIDS patients who had experienced one bout of *pneumocystis* pneumonia were divided into two groups. One group received AZT, while the other control group received placebo pills that contained no drug. The physical states of all of the subjects were then monitored on a regular basis. After the study was in progress for six months, the results showed markedly better survival of the group taking AZT than the control group. In fact, the results were so striking that the investigators terminated the trial early and administered AZT to the control patients as well. Withholding the drug would have been unethical at that point. These studies led to approval of AZT for therapy in AIDS. Other studies are now in progress to test different administration routines for AZT and its use in other AIDS-related conditions (see Chapter 5). Other possible antiviral drugs (Chapters 4 and 5) have been tested as well.

Table 6–5
EFFECT OF AZIDOTHYMIDINE TREATMENT ON SURVIVAL OF AIDS AND ARC PATIENTS*

Treatment	Number of Subjects	Number of Deaths	Percent Deaths
None (Placebo pills)	97	19	19.6
AZT	124	1	0.8

*The subjects were in the study an average of 16 to 17 weeks. The study was intended to last 24 weeks (6 months), but it was terminated early, once the dramatic effect of AZT treatment became evident. All subjects were offered AZT at that time. These data are taken from the report of the first large-scale test of AZT (Fishl et al., New England J. Med. 317:185 [1987]).

AIDS AROUND THE WORLD

AIDS in Africa

As mentioned previously, AIDS is a major health problem in sub-Saharan Africa. The disease is centered in countries of central Africa, including Zaire, Kenya, Uganda, Zambia, and Rwanda. In contrast to the distribution of cases in North America and Europe, HIV infection is distributed equally among men and women, and epidemiology reflects the fact that a predominant mode of transmission is heterosexual intercourse. Other modes of transmission may include blood transfusions, injections with reused needles, and procedures that involve scraping the skin with surgical knives (scarifications). The epidemic probably spread along truck routes through central Africa, and female prostitutes have been important reservoirs for the infection. The AIDS epidemic is mostly concentrated in cities and urban areas and is much lower in rural areas. As in North America and Europe, the spread of HIV infection in Africa is a recent phenomenon, mostly occurring in the 1980s.

The extent of HIV infection in sub-Saharan Africa is alarmingly high. For example, as many as 90 percent of female prostitutes in Nairobi, Kenya, are HIV infected today. In 1985–1986, 18 percent of men visiting venereal disease clinics in Nairobi were seropositive for HIV, and the percentage has rapidly climbed since then. As many as 25 percent of the sexually active populations of some cities in Rwanda may be infected. There may be 10 million HIV-infected individuals in Africa, many of whom will probably progress to AIDS and eventually die. This will have devastating social and economic impact on these countries and may reach the proportions of some of the ancient epidemics described in Chapter 2.

Another virus related to HIV has also been discovered in Africa. The original HIV that is associated with the great majority of AIDS cases is called *HIV-1* (see Chapter 4). The new virus is called *HIV-2* and is predominantly found in countries along the west African coast, such as Senegal and the Ivory Coast. Molecular biological experiments tell us that HIV-1 and HIV-2 are closely related but distinct viruses that evolved from a common ancestor hundreds or thousands of years ago. HIV-2 also causes AIDS, although there are some indications that it is less able to cause disease than HIV-1.

It is interesting that the virus that is most closely related to HIV-2 is not HIV-1, but a lentivirus found in sooty mangabey monkeys (simian immunodeficiency virus or SIV_{SM}). SIV_{SM} does not cause disease in sooty mangabeys.

The existence of HIV-2 raises a problem since the standard HIV-1 ELISA tests will not detect HIV-2 antibodies. Thus, the standard HIV test will not detect individuals infected with HIV-2. So far in North America, few cases of HIV-2 infection have been found. However, it may be important to screen blood supplies and individuals for HIV-2 infection as well, in order to avoid undetected contamination or infections.

AIDS in Asia

While the largest number of HIV infections is presently in Africa, the world region where HIV infection is increasing most rapidly on a percentage basis is Asia. Once HIV enters a high-risk population, it can spread extremely rapidly, if proper precautions (e.g., safer sex practices, injection drug precautions) are not taken. Until recently, infection rates in most Asian countries have been relatively low. However, HIV infection has begun to spread rapidly among commercial sex workers and injection drug users in India and Thailand. In these countries, heterosexual sex and injection drug use are the major routes of infection. While the overall infection levels in the general population for these countries is still rather low (about 1 percent but climbing), the levels of infection and the rates of increase in the high-risk populations are striking. For instance, in one six-month period (January to July 1988), the percentage of HIV-positive injection drug users monitored by one Bangkok hospital climbed from 1 percent to more than 30 percent. In 1991, 50 percent of patients attending sexually transmitted disease clinics in Bombay were HIV positive. It is estimated that there may be 700,000 to 1 million infected people in India today, and that number is increasing unchecked. As in other parts of the world, the concern is that without intervention, these infections will spread into other populations in these countries, leading to the situations that confront many sub-Saharan African countries today.

It is important to note that these figures represent HIV-infected individuals (detected by the antibody test described in Chapter 4), not AIDS cases. Since most of these infected individuals acquired the virus relatively recently, most have not begun to show signs of illness yet. However, we can predict that within a few years, the number of AIDS cases in these countries will soar. Since there are not very many cases of frank AIDS in these countries yet, it is easy for the general public (and politicians) to ignore or downplay the problem for the time being.

The worldwide nature of HIV infection makes it a very important public health problem. No continents or countries are safe from infection, and the virus can spread rapidly (and undetected) once it enters a high-risk group. Public health officials predict that there will be 45 million to 110 million cases of HIV infection worldwide by the year 2000, if current rates of spread continue. The majority of these cases are likely to be in Asia.

Chapter 7
Modes of HIV Transmission and Personal Risk Factors

BIOLOGICAL BASES OF HIV TRANSMISSION

- Sources of Infectious HIV
- Stability of HIV
- Targets for HIV Infection

MODES OF HIV TRANSMISSION

- No Association with HIV Transmission: Casual Contact
- Activities Associated with HIV Transmission
  Perinatal Transmission between an Infected Mother and Her Gestating Infant
  Transmission from an HIV-Infected Source to the Bloodstream
  Intimate Sexual Contact with an HIV-Infected Person

In previous chapters, we analyzed how the AIDS virus operates at the cellular level and at the organism level. Now our focus shifts to the interorganism level. In this chapter, we will look specifically at the question of how HIV is transmitted from person to person. Because there currently is no cure for AIDS once an individual has contracted the disease, preventing the transmission of HIV from person to person is critical. Consequently, in this chapter, we shall consider risk factors for HIV transmission and discuss ways of reducing these risk factors.

The evidence for assigning risks to different levels of activities comes from two main sources: theoretical biological considerations and empirical epidemiological data, bolstered by laboratory data. Theoretical analysis considers the biological plausibility of HIV transmission for particular activities based on the presence or absence of substances containing HIV and of receptors for these substances. For example, we know that HIV is not present in someone's exhaled breath; consequently, on the basis of theoretical analysis alone, we would assign little risk to breathing the air in the same room with a person with AIDS.

Theoretical analysis can be used to make predictions about no-, low-, or high-risk activities. These ultimately can be tested by empirical epidemiological data, the other main source of evidence for our risk judgments in this chapter. To continue the example above, epidemiological data from the sample of individuals who have lived with people with AIDS provides corroborating evidence that breathing the same air does not spread HIV (see Chapter 6). Because epidemiological data indicate no AIDS incidence among family and friends who have simply lived with people with AIDS, and because of the biological implausibility, we can confidently state that breathing the same air is not a risk factor.

Typically, it is those activities with a high biological plausibility of HIV transmission that are carefully investigated with epidemiological studies. We saw one example of this in the last chapter. Anal receptive sexual activity has a high biological plausibility of HIV transmission, and the evidence from epidemiological studies discussed in Chapter 6 provides corroborative evidence that this behavior is in fact strongly associated with HIV infection.

In addition, epidemiological evidence can provide the initial evidence that certain activities are or are not associated with HIV infection risk. At the outset of the AIDS epidemic, for instance, it was epidemiological studies that led to the identification of likely modes of HIV transmission. This, in part, guided subsequent biological laboratory work, aided in the theoretical understanding of AIDS, and resulted in the isolation of HIV.

We should remember one aspect of epidemiological information at the outset of our discussion of risk and risk factors. Epidemiological studies have identified certain groups of individuals who are overrepresented in the population of those with AIDS: in particular, gay and bisexual men and injection drug users make up a large percentage of those with AIDS. There is nothing about being gay, bisexual, or an injection drug user which, by itself, leads to HIV infection and AIDS. Rather, these groups of individuals are, on average, more likely to undertake certain behaviors that have a high biological plausibility of HIV transmission. In addition, because of the greater prevalence of HIV infection among people in these groups, the likelihood of transmission is increased if the necessary and sufficient behaviors for HIV transmission occur.

Consider, for example, two cases: a homosexual man (Jim) who has unprotected anal sex with another homosexual man, and a heterosexual woman (Susan) who has unprotected vaginal sex with a heterosexual man. Assume that neither Jim nor Susan is HIV positive. In each case, Jim and Susan are involved in behaviors that have a high biological plausibility for HIV transmission. The important and unknown factor, then, is the HIV status of their partners. On the sole basis of *average* HIV infection rates, which are higher among gay men as a group than among heterosexual men as a group, Jim is at more risk than Susan. However, without complete data on their partner's HIV status and sexual history, neither Jim nor Susan can be certain of their risk for this particular sexual encounter. The safest approach, as we shall see below, is to avoid unprotected anal or vaginal intercourse.

Before we consider the risks of particular behaviors, however, we need to understand the biological bases of HIV transmission, including such issues as the primary sources of HIV within an infected person, the stability of the virus in moving between individuals, and the targets for infection in an uninfected individual.

BIOLOGICAL BASES OF HIV TRANSMISSION

In infected people, infectious HIV is present only in cells and human body fluids. Despite its devastating effects within the body, the virus is actually quite fragile in the external environment and dies quickly when exposed to room temperature and air conditions. In fact, very special laboratory conditions are needed to grow HIV outside the human body. It is important to remember this fact because it is easy to assume mistakenly that a disease as deadly as AIDS must be caused by an agent that is tremendously strong and sturdy. People's fears of the disease, combined with their lack of knowledge and mistaken impressions about epidemics, can cause them to view HIV in an anthropomorphic way—almost like a living, breathing enemy capable of thought and devastating action. Instead, the reality of HIV outside the body is much different: a fragile virus that loses infectivity quickly.

Sources of Infectious HIV

In an infected individual, HIV is present in certain cells, as well as in bodily fluids and secretions, many of which also contain these cells. In terms of cells, macrophages and T_{helper} lymphocytes are susceptible to infection by HIV, as described in Chapter 4.

Macrophages may be the long-term reservoirs of HIV in infected individuals since they are not killed by the virus. Macrophages circulate through the bloodstream, and they also are found in all mucosal linings of the body, such as the internal urogenital surface of the vagina and penis, the lining of the anus, lungs, and throat. Another kind of cell that can be infected with HIV is the Langerhans cell of the skin.

Among people who test positive for HIV, the virus is not found consistently in all body fluids and products. Furthermore, in body fluids where HIV is regularly found, it occurs in different concentrations at different times. Nonetheless, we can place the body fluids and products into three groups based on the degree of association between body fluids/products and HIV infection. These groupings reflect differences among body fluids/products in their general concentrations of infectious HIV or HIV-infected cells and in the amount of relative exposure a typical individual might experience. Table 7–1 lists these groupings.

Researchers have developed methods to test for HIV and estimate the amounts of infectious virus present in various body fluids and secretions (see Chapter 4). HIV can be isolated relatively easily from blood, semen, and vaginal/cervical secretions (including menstrual fluid). When blood and semen are examined closely, the great majority of HIV is associated with infected

---

Table 7–1

DEGREE OF ASSOCIATION BETWEEN HIV INFECTION AND DIFFERENT BODY FLUIDS AND PRODUCTS

Group 1: Very High Association

| Blood | Semen | Vaginal/Cervical Secretion (incl. menstrual fluid) |

Group 2: High Association

Breast Milk

Group 3: Low or No Association

| Saliva | Tears | Perspiration/Sweat |
| Urine | Feces | |

cells (mostly macrophages) present in these fluids. In blood, if the cells are removed, low levels of HIV are present in the cell-free serum. It has also been isolated from breast milk. With much greater difficulty, the virus has, on occasion, been isolated from saliva, tears, and urine. It has not been isolated from perspiration and feces. The current scientific view is that body fluids and products *other* than blood, semen, vaginal/cervical secretions, and breast milk contain so little if any HIV that they are not of major importance in HIV transmission between individuals.

Blood and semen are of greatest concern when we consider HIV transmission because of another factor: These are the most infectious fluids to which a potential target individual might be exposed during activities typically associated with HIV transmission (sexual behavior or injection drug use). These issues are covered in detail later in this chapter. The relative HIV infectivity of different body fluids and products can be explained in another way, using biological considerations. The fluids and products listed in Table 7–1 differ in the amount of live cells they contain. Blood, semen, vaginal/cervical secretions, and breast milk contain high numbers of live cells. The other body fluids and products (saliva, tears, perspiration, urine, and feces) are completely or nearly completely free of live cells (although they may contain nonhuman cells, such as bacteria). Since live infected cells produce HIV, we would expect fluids with live cells to pose the greatest risks for HIV transmission.

Stability of HIV

For transmission of HIV infection to occur, infectious virus must survive long enough to pass to a susceptible person and infect target cells. The HIV virus particle (see Chapter 4) is actually a very fragile one, as discussed above. As a result, the virus quickly becomes inactivated when exposed to drying effects of air or light. It is also quickly inactivated by contact with soap and water.

As mentioned above, much of the infectious HIV is associated with cells (macrophages). In blood or semen, cells will maintain infectious HIV as long as they themselves are alive. Thus, intravenous transfusions or sexual intercourse involving HIV-infected individuals efficiently transmits infection, since live cells are passed. On the other hand, if blood or semen is allowed to dry, the cells die quite quickly and the HIV infectivity is lost.

These facts about the stability of HIV, combined with the facts about likely sources of HIV infection, explain why casual contact with people with AIDS does not result in the spread of HIV infection (see Chapter 6 and below).

Targets for HIV Infection

At the cellular level, HIV infection requires the presence of virus receptors on the cell surface. As described in Chapter 4, the receptor for HIV is the CD4 surface protein, which is only present on T $_{helper}$ lymphocytes and macrophages. Thus, these are the predominant cells that become infected in a susceptible individual. These cells are most abundant in the blood. Consequently, activities that introduce infectious HIV, either as infected cells or free virus, into the blood of an uninfected individual will potentially result in infection. For example, sexual intercourse can result in damage or tears (sometimes microscopic) of the mucosal linings of the male or female genital tracts or of the anus. These tears can allow passage of blood or semen into the circulatory system of the uninfected individual. In addition, as described above, macrophages are also present at the mucosal surfaces of the anus and genital tract, and they potentially can be infected directly without the necessity of virus entry into the bloodstream.

There is another potential target for HIV infection: the oral cavity and the throat. Like the genital tract and the anus, the throat has a mucosal lining that contains macrophages. In certain sexual activities, such as oral sex, semen is exchanged orally from one person to another. Consequently, there is the theoretical potential for infection. The epidemiological reality, however, is that oral sex is not a primary mode of transmission of HIV, as we shall see below. The explanation for this may be that there is less physical trauma associated with oral sex or that chemical and physiological features of the oral cavity reduce the efficiency of transmission. This case demonstrates the need to combine theoretical predictions from biology with epidemiological data about actual incidence rates in order to understand fully the risks of actual HIV transmission. It is this topic to which we now turn.

MODES OF HIV TRANSMISSION

We are now ready to analyze the modes of HIV transmission from person to person and the relative risks associated with different modes. In making our assessment of risk, we will rely on both the plausibility of HIV transmission, based on theoretical biological analysis, and the empirical facts associating documented HIV transmission with various modes, drawn from epidemiological studies. Together, these two sources of information permit us to categorize activities and behaviors according to the degree of their association with HIV infection.

No Association with HIV Transmission: Casual Contact

Because HIV is so fragile outside the body, transmission requires *direct* contact of two substances: fluid containing infectious HIV from an infected person and susceptible cells (usually via the bloodstream) of another person. Because of the absence of this type of direct contact, a large group of interpersonal activities and behaviors, generally referred to as *casual contact*, have no measured association with HIV transmission (see Chapter 6) and therefore pose no risk for HIV infection.

What do we mean by casual contact? This includes all types of ordinary, everyday, nonsexual contacts between and among people. Shaking hands, hugging, kissing, sharing eating utensils, sharing towels or napkins, using the same telephone, and using the same toilet seat are a few examples of casual contact. It is impossible to list all types of casual contact here, but we can analyze or make predictions about others, keeping in mind the need for direct contact with body fluids containing infectious HIV. For example, consider the possibilities of waterborne or airborne transmission. Because HIV is quickly inactivated outside the body, it cannot survive in the open air or in water. Consequently, we would predict that there is no risk in sharing the

Table 7–2
MODES OF HIV TRANSMISSION

1. Birth: Perinatal transmission between an infected mother and her gestating infant.
2. Blood: Transmission from an HIV-infected source to the bloodstream.
3. Sex: Intimate sexual contact with an HIV-infected person.

same physical space with a person with AIDS or swimming in the same pool. Epidemiological evidence supports this conclusion: There is no measured risk of transmission.

Activities Associated with HIV Transmission

HIV transmission needs to occur directly between HIV-tainted fluid from an infected person into the bloodstream or onto a mucosal lining of another person. Epidemiological data point to three modes of HIV transmission from person to person: via birth, via blood, or via sex. For most people, the last mode of transmission—via sex—is the most likely, and we discuss it at length below. First, however, we will briefly discuss the other two modes. These are listed in Table 7–2 and discussed below.

Perinatal Transmission between an Infected Mother and Her Gestating Infant

This mode of HIV transmission brings together a source of HIV (in the bloodstream of an HIV-infected woman) and a potential target (the bloodstream of a developing fetus) in a protected environment (the mother's body). The mother's and child's bloodstreams are separated by the placenta, which prevents exchange of cells but not of nutrients. But during the third trimester of pregnancy, small tears sometimes occur in the placenta, which can lead to entry of cells from the mother's bloodstream into the child's. In addition, during birth, the child frequently comes into close contact with the mother's blood due to the bleeding associated with delivery. Current statistics indicate that there is about a 30 percent chance that a child of an infected mother will be infected.

Transmission from an HIV-Infected Source to the
Bloodstream

This mode of transmission relates to receiving blood or
blood products. This can occur in two main ways: receiving a
transfusion of HIV-infected blood or injecting oneself with an
HIV-infected syringe (either accidentally or incidentally).

Receiving a transfusion of HIV-infected blood   Since a
transfusion involves placing foreign blood or blood products directly into the recipient's bloodstream, the necessary conditions
for HIV transmission are present: direct contact of potentially
infected fluid with susceptible cells in the recipient. Prior to 1985,
when screening of the blood supply for HIV by the antibody test
was begun (see Chapter 4), the sufficient condition for contracting AIDS was present: HIV-infected blood for transfusion. Even
then, however, the risk was low that the blood or blood product
involved in a transfusion was infected—except for hemophiliacs
who required a clotting factor extracted from the blood of many
different donors. Now, this sufficient condition is very unlikely.

It is estimated that 18 million units of blood components
are transfused per year in the United States. In 1984, the year before antibody test screening of the blood supply was begun, the
risk of receiving HIV-infected blood was 40 out of 100,000. Now,
the risk is 2.25 out of 100,000. Why is there still some risk? This
occurs because the screening tests are not perfect and because of
the possibility that detectable antibodies have not yet developed
in a recently infected donor. Compared with the risk of dying
from the condition for which a person is hospitalized and requires a transfusion (that is 40 out of 100 or 40,000 out of
100,000), the risk of receiving HIV-infected blood during a transfusion is about 15,500 times less.

Blood donation centers have developed methods to reduce
the risk even further. In addition to routine screening using the
tests discussed in Chapter 4, centers have developed information
campaigns that discourage blood donation from those who might
be infected. New procedures also have been established to permit
donors, particularly those who may feel pressured during a work-

associated blood drive, to indicate confidentially that their blood should not be used. The American Red Cross blood donation offices give all blood donors a special card describing a procedure that must be followed by all potential donors. The card lists nine groups of people who should not give blood, then describes a confidential procedure that all donors must follow, involving barcode labels indicating "transfuse" or "do not transfuse." People in one of the nine groups (e.g., drug users, men who have had sex with men since 1977) are to remove the "do not transfuse" bar code tag and place it on another card. Those not in one of the listed groups remove the "transfuse" bar code tag and place it on the card. To the casual observer, the bar code tags are identical but not to the optical scanner, which later identifies the blood to be rejected. As these procedures become routinely accepted by staff and donors, the risk of receiving infected blood or blood products from a transfusion will become even smaller.

Before we conclude this section, it is important to note two points. First, we have been analyzing the potential risks of receiving a blood transfusion, not of donating blood. There are no risks of HIV transmission from donating blood. The donor's blood is the only potential source of HIV in this situation: If there is no HIV in that blood, there is no other source of the virus. Second, receipt of an organ transplant is a possible source of HIV, were the organ donor HIV-infected. Like blood donations, organ donations are tested for HIV, so the risk is quite small.*

Injecting oneself with HIV-infected blood   There are two ways that HIV-infected blood in needles could lead to transmission: when needles are shared during intravenous (IV) drug use and through accidental needle sticks between HIV-infected individuals and health workers. Both are discussed below.

In the case of IV drug use, the two necessary elements are present: infected blood and direct injection of that blood into the bloodstream. During the process of injecting the drug, an individual draws blood into the syringe to be sure that the needle is in a vein. Infected blood, then, can be mixed with the drug solu-

*Sperm donations also could be HIV-infected and are screened for HIV.

tion. If the syringe is passed to another individual and inserted into his or her body, infected blood from the previous person can be passed into the bloodstream as part of the drug solution.

At first, this mode of transmission may appear contradictory, in that HIV is taken *outside* the body first, then passed to another individual. This occurs, however, in the special context of a protective container—the closed confines of the syringe—where blood cells and virus are not exposed to the environment. In addition, it is generally done in a very short time, usually within seconds or, at most, minutes. Consequently, the blood cells remain alive and, with them, the HIV.

Prevention of this mode of transmission involves breaking the link between individuals via the syringe. IV drug users are encouraged first not to share needles. Some cities provide free sterile needles so that limited syringe availability is not an issue. Alternatively, IV drug users are encouraged to clean their needles between administrations, using a bleach solution.

The other mode of HIV infection is accidental needle sticks among health workers. On occasion, health workers, in emergency situations or in the process of medical laboratory work with HIV-infected people, have accidentally stuck themselves with potentially contaminated needles. A 1991 report presented data on the 1,989 U.S. health care workers who received needle sticks with HIV-contaminated blood (out of the approximately 100,000 needle sticks that occur each year in the United States). Only six became HIV infected. In total (through January 1992), the U.S. Centers for Disease Control had documented 40 cases of health-care workers who became infected with HIV due to needle sticks, mucous membrane exposures, and blood exposure. Of these 40 people, only three have developed full-blown AIDS, one of whom has died.

The most common risk of HIV infection for health-care workers is an accidental needle stick. As the data presented above show, however, the risk is quite low. Nonetheless, the risk does exist, and health workers have been advised to wear gloves during clinical procedures and to discard used needles directly rather than recap before discarding. In addition, new needles have been designed that make accidental sticks more difficult.

Intimate Sexual Contact with an HIV-Infected
Person

For most people in the general public, this mode of transmission is the most likely source of HIV infection. The risk differs, however, depending one the particular sexual practice, the
frequency of the practice, and the HIV status of a sexual partner.
We cannot, therefore, categorize particular sexual practices with
certainty in terms of their HIV risk. The degree of risk of any particular sexual behavior for a particular individual differs from
person to person. Individual risk assessment, however, is usually
a difficult task, based on incomplete and sometimes unknowable
data (e.g., the HIV status of a new sexual partner).

To make this task somewhat easier, we can discuss what
we know from the theoretical and epidemiological perspectives.
Together, the data from these perspectives complement each
other and provide useful information in judging the relative risk
of various sexual practices.

From the theoretical perspective, we know that we need two
critical elements together: HIV-contaminated body fluid (in particular, blood or semen) and direct contact of this fluid with a target site. The riskiest sexual practices, therefore, would be those in
which HIV-infected blood or semen from an infected person comes
in immediate and direct contact with the bloodstream or mucous
membranes of another person. These practices include vaginal intercourse between a man and a woman, anal intercourse between
a man and a woman, and anal intercourse between two men. In all
of these practices, semen from the man is deposited into vagina or
anus—both sites of macrophages or other susceptible cells and
also sites where small tears frequently occur during intercourse.

At the other end of the spectrum, the least risky sexual practices would be those where HIV-infected blood or semen does not
usually come into contact with target sites. These practices would
include masturbation by a male onto unbroken skin of a partner
and dry kissing (closed-mouth kissing). In the case of male masturbation, while potentially infected semen is present, a target site
is not—unbroken skin of a partner. In the case of dry kissing, neither blood nor semen is usually present and saliva of HIV-infected
people has been shown to contain little or no HIV.

On this spectrum of risk, we can anchor the ends of potentially risky sexual behaviors but cannot precisely anchor other groups of sexual practices or consider every possible case that could arise. For example, what if two people are dry kissing and one has a cut on her lip: Is there a risk of HIV infection? Or, what if a man masturbates onto chapped skin: Is there a risk of HIV infection? The answer to both questions is "possibly." Here is where the epidemiological evidence is useful.

We know that, across groups of people, those who frequently engage in particular sexual practices are more likely to become HIV infected. The three sexual practices listed above at the riskiest end of the spectrum of risk (vaginal intercourse with an HIV-infected person without a condom, anal intercourse with an HIV-infected person without a condom) have been shown, through epidemiological data, to be highly associated with HIV infection. The two practices from the least-risky end of the spectrum (dry kissing between an HIV-infected person and masturbation by an HIV-infected male onto the unbroken skin of a partner) have not been shown, through epidemiological data, to be associated with HIV infection.

Epidemiological data also provide clues to the relative infectivity of other sexual practices. Wet kissing (open-mouth kissing with exchange of saliva) has not been shown to be associated with HIV transmission. This makes sense from a biological perspective too, since we know that saliva of an HIV-infected person contains little, if any, HIV. Oral sex performed on an HIV-infected man or woman by either a woman or a man has not been strongly associated with HIV transmission, although there are some reported cases of transmission via this sexual practice. From a biological perspective, we can see why this might be the case, if the HIV-infected semen is deposited in the mouth and throat or possibly into the bloodstream via small tears in the mouth. Still, there must be other chemical or physiological factors (e.g., the acidity of the mouth) that provide some barrier to HIV transmission, since the epidemiological data do not show oral sex to be highly associated with HIV transmission.

From our analysis of the relative risk of various sexual practices based on biological and epidemiological considerations, we can not only place the sexual practices on the spectrum of HIV risk but also see ways to reduce the risks of all sexual practices that could involve some risk. Abstinence from sexual relations clearly reduces the risk of transmission to zero: no source and no target. Abstinence, however, is not a realistic option for many sexually active people. These people can choose to have sexual relations of the least risky types. If they choose riskier sexual practices, they can reduce the risks by placing barriers between potential sources of HIV infection and potential targets. For example, they can use condoms during vaginal and anal intercourse to reduce the risk of HIV infection by containing potentially infected semen within the condom and preventing its contact with target sites in the vagina or anus. Condom use during oral sex on a man also provides a barrier between potentially infectious semen and the target sites in the mouth and throat. During oral sex on a woman, a dental dam (a 3–4-inch square piece of latex) placed over the vagina also provides a barrier for source-to-target-site contact.

These protective methods are not 100 percent effective. Condoms can have holes and can leak; however, this is not at all frequent. Studies are regularly done on condom reliability, and condom manufacturers pay close attention to quality control procedures. Properly used, condoms provide a good measure of protection for most people. A condom should be fresh and made of latex (not of natural products). The condom must be placed on the man's erect penis prior to any penetration, since pre-ejaculatory fluid has been shown to be HIV infected in an HIV-infected individual. Space should be left in the tip of the condom for the semen which will soon be ejaculated, and the condom should be unrolled completely to the base of the erect penis. If a lubricant is used during intercourse, it should be water based, not a grease- or oil-based lubricant, which destroys latex. For even more protection, condoms or lubricants with nonoxynol-9, a spermicide that kills HIV, should be used. The condom must stay in place at the base of the penis until the penis is withdrawn from the vagina or anus; this is best done before the man's erection fades and the penis is flaccid and separated from the stretched condom.

Each person has to analyze his or her own sexual practices and take the precautions necessary for protection from HIV. The guidelines described above for self-protection are similar to those advocated by the U.S. Surgeon General, the U.S. Centers for Disease Control, and many local AIDS prevention programs. The final decisions on individual risk assessment and management are made differently by each of us. Although we will never have all the data we need to make perfect decisions, we can make use of information from biological and epidemiological studies to assess the risks of various sexual practices. These assessments are best made prior to sexual activity, when our thinking is less affected by volatile emotions and judgment-confusing substances (alcohol or drugs), which are sometimes associated with sexual behavior for some people. Because sexual activity usually involves two people, it is necessary to think about HIV risk assessment and make decisions on HIV-risk management *together* with your sexual partner *prior* to sexual activity. Then, for those who choose to have sexual relations, they will be ready to enjoy the sexual experience more, knowing that they have taken the necessary precautions to lower the risk of HIV transmission.

Chapter 8

Individual Assessments
of HIV Risk

We begin now to look at HIV and AIDS from the individual's perspective. In this and the next two chapters, we will address questions such as these: How do individuals assess their own risk of HIV? What contribution can the HIV antibody test make to this assessment? What factors affect individuals' knowledge, attitudes, intentions, and behaviors related to HIV and AIDS? How can these factors be incorporated into HIV and AIDS prevention programs? How do individuals—both those with HIV and AIDS and those who are not infected—live with the realities of AIDS? In this chapter, we focus on the first two questions related to assessing HIV risk. Following an introduction to the general process of individual decision making, we will consider two main topics: the general issue of individual risk assessment and the specific issue of HIV testing.

INTRODUCTION TO INDIVIDUAL DECISION MAKING AND ACTION

Each of us is constantly making decisions that affect our actions. Many of these decisions are minor ones and relatively unimportant ("What will I have for breakfast?"), but others are major and have significant consequences ("What job will I take?"). Still other decisions may seem minor at the time ("Do I wear a condom if I have sex?"), but they can have important outcomes (in this instance, decreasing or increasing the risk of HIV transmission). In all of these cases, there is a general model that underlies each.

There are four basic steps in the model, ordered temporally:

1. knowledge
2. attitude
3. intention
4. behavior

The "knowledge" step involves information collection, synthesis, and weighing. The "attitude" step condenses this information into a conclusion. The "intention" step involves a readiness to take action, and the "behavior" step is the action actually taken.

This is a simplified model intended to separate the parts of the decision-making and action process so that we can understand the factors affecting each step related to HIV and AIDS. This chapter will focus primarily on the first two steps for individuals making assessment of their own HIV risk. The next chapter will expand the picture to the other steps. There are different factors that affect the four steps; an individual's weighing of information in the "knowledge" step, for example, is affected by different considerations than his or her actions in the "behavior" step.

In the case of HIV and AIDS, the decision-making process is a particularly complex one at the early stages because of the probabilistic nature of HIV risk information. In the following section, we discuss several factors that affect individuals' assessment of information such as that related to HIV transmission.

RISK ASSESSMENT

Consciously or unconsciously, each of us is making risk assessments throughout our day as part of our decision making. Should I choose the salad or the french fries with my sandwich, knowing that the salad is better for me? If I select the salad, do I choose the tasty but fatty dressing (knowing that extra calories and fat are not good for my heart and arteries) or do I decide on a little lemon juice instead (knowing that it has almost no calories and fat—but also less taste)? Likewise, confronted with a need to take action related to our risk of contracting HIV, we have to weigh information about risks before we make decisions. Karen and I are going to have sex: Could she have the HIV virus? Do I have the virus? What are the HIV transmission potentials for different sexual acts? How do different prevention measures (such as using a condom) affect the HIV transmission potentials? Much of this risk information is probabilistic and therefore has to be considered in special ways. What is probabilistic information and what are the "special ways" used to consider it?

Probabilistic information is information containing an estimate related to an issue or topic. The estimate may be about likelihood, frequency, or prevalence. For example, the weather bureau's announcement that there is a "40 percent chance of showers" is probabilistic information. Another example would be the statement that 1 in 200 college students (or, stated a different way, 0.5 percent) test positive for the HIV virus. These statements provide some information but do not tell us exactly what we would like to know in each case in order to make a decision and take action.

For instance, knowing that there is a 40 percent chance of showers does not directly lead to a clear conclusion that we should take an umbrella or cancel our tennis game. In this example, the more extreme the probability (for example, a 5 percent or a 95 percent chance of rain), the clearer the situation becomes, and the easier it is for us to use this probabilistic information in making conclusions and decisions.

In the case of the probabilistic information about the prevalence of HIV among college students, we face a different kind of situation. The probabilistic information provides knowledge about a general, large group but not about particular individuals in a particular subgroup. The "1 in 200" figure tells us that, over many different groups of college students, about 1 in 200 will test positive for HIV. It does not mean that, if we draw one group of 200 college students, we will find exactly one who is HIV positive. In this particular group, we might find none who is HIV positive or we might find four who are. But, if we draw a series of groups of 200 college students, from different campuses with different students, we should find the "1 in 200" figure to be generally true. (Indeed, this is basically how the figure was discovered.)

Let's take the college student example one step further. The risk assessment facing a particular college student (say,

Marc) who is considering sexual contact with another college student (say, Amy) is whether Amy is HIV positive. The "1 in 200" figure gives Marc only a very limited amount of information and cannot tell him whether Amy is HIV positive. Marc must also consider other probabilistic information: the degree of risk for HIV transmission associated with particular sexual practices and the degree of protection against HIV transmission afforded by various products (condoms, spermicidal foams). Some of this latter probabilistic information is not even available in numerical form. For example, in the last chapter, we talked about "least risky" or "most risky" sexual practices; we cannot assign percentages or proportions to particular practices or even to groups of practices beyond these general characterizations.

What is Marc (our hypothetical risk assessor) to do in making conclusions from all of this information about what will happen between him and Amy? This question moves us to the issue of "special ways" to consider probabilistic information. There are two main ways probabilistic information is weighed: according to a normative judgment model or according to a subjective probability model. The normative model is the way scientists weigh probability information in reaching decisions; whereas, the subjective probability model is the way lay people weigh probability information.

Normative Model

In the normative model, probability information is weighted according to statistical rules to reach conclusions. A detailed understanding of these statistical rules is not necessary for our purpose here. What is important, however, is a general understanding of how the normative model is applied by scientists, and this can be conveyed by an example.[1]

In this illustration of the normative model, the decision to be made is this: What is the occupation of the person described in the following sentences? "Steve is very shy and withdrawn, invariably helpful, but with little interest in people or in the world of reality. A meek and tidy soul, he has a need for order and structure, and a passion for detail." The list of possibilities includes farmer, salesman, airline pilot, librarian, and physician. What is Steve's occupation?

In making his or her decision, a scientist using the normative model would consider the base-rate frequency of each occupation in the population. If one occupation is much more common in the general population than the others, the likelihood is that Steve is from that population and the best choice would be that occupation. There are, for instance, many more farmers than librarians, so "farmer" would be the normative model choice.

There are other normative model rules that can come into play, as relevant, when scientists make decisions. One other rule that the reader may be familiar with is the independence of random or chance events. If we toss a coin four times, each toss is independent and the outcome of the next toss (heads or tails) is independent of the previous toss and all earlier tosses. If the first three tosses of the coin gave heads, heads, and heads, the scientist using the normative model would predict an equal chance of either heads or tails, since each toss is independent. (Put another way, the coin cannot "know" the outcomes of the previous tosses.)

In each of these examples, the reader may have made his or her own decisions about Steve's occupation or the outcome of the fourth coin toss—and these decisions likely were not what the normative model would predict. This is common (many of our students think Steve is a librarian—even with the additional information about the base-rate frequencies—and that the fourth toss will be tails.) These conclusions are also understandable and should not be labeled "irrational." There is a set of rules being used, but these rules come from a different model: the subjective probability model.

Subjective Probability Model

Most of us do not and cannot use the normative model for our decision making. We do not know all the statistical rules and, even if we knew all the rules, we do not and cannot have all the data, since probability data can keep changing. (As an example, think about the variations in the weather reports we receive over the day; what was a 40 percent chance of rain in the morning may be a 60 percent chance by mid-afternoon.)

Judgment Heuristics

The rules most of us use to make decisions based on probabilistic information are known as "judgment heuristics." These are rules-of-thumb, identified in a variety of research studies, which provide shortcuts in processing probabilistic information. We consider three of these heuristics: representativeness, availability, and anchoring.

Representativeness   One general decision-making rule-of-thumb that most of us typically use to assess probabilistic information is representativeness. We conclude that one item or object is representative of another to the degree that the two items or objects are similar. Then, if similarity is high, we generalize from what we know—or think we know—about probabilities.

Think back to the example of matching the description of Steve ("... very shy and withdrawn ... little interest in people ... a meek and tidy soul ... ") and his likely occupation (farmer, salesman, airline pilot, librarian, or physician). Using representativeness, most people compare the details of the description to the stereotype of a librarian, note a high similarity, and conclude that Steve is a librarian.

The representative heuristic can be a useful shortcut, but it also can lead to errors in judgment because it ignores factors that are relevant to judgments of probability. In discussing the same example of Steve, we noted that scientists (using the normative model) would consider factors such as the base-rate of different occupations in the population. A lay person using the representative heuristic does not consider base rates and therefore can be misled if, as in this example, there are many more farmers than librarians in the general population. Even if lay people are informed about the base-rate information, they do not necessarily make major adjustments in their decisions. The power of the representativeness heuristic can be strong.

In some cases, then, the representativeness rule-of-thumb helps us make decisions quickly and relatively accurately. In other cases, however, this decision-making shortcut can get us into trouble. Consider an example involving Nancy, a college student, who is estimating the risk of contracting HIV from her fellow students. In her judgment, she compares the similarity (that is, the representativeness) of her peer group and two groups she understands to have high HIV infection rates: male homosexuals and IV drug users. She sees little similarity and concludes that the risk must be low. In addition, she compares her fellow students and the general population, a group that has a very low HIV infection rate, and sees many similarities. Consequently, she concludes that her risk is very low.

In fact, the HIV infection rate among college students (about 1 in 200) is considered very high by the U.S. Centers for Disease Control and Prevention. Nancy's conclusion, using the representativeness heuristic, that her risk is low would underestimate the risk of HIV infection from her fellow students. It is important to understand that Nancy is not intentionally distorting the data and making irrational decisions. Instead, she is making comparisons that seem appropriate to her, then using the representativeness heuristic to generalize about probabilities of HIV infection rates. (There may be cases where additional factors are present—for instance, a strong emotional factor—which may distort the subjective probability assessment. The influence of some of these other factors are considered later in this chapter and in the next chapter.)

Consider another example related to HIV and AIDS where decisions made on the basis of the representativeness heuristic could lead to problems of a different sort, this time in the overestimate of HIV transmission risk. Miguel works as a clerk at a health clinic that has some HIV positive clients. He is considering his degree of HIV risk from his contact with these clients. He believes that viruses, like the common cold, can be spread by casual contact (kissing someone with a cold, breathing the same air after someone with a cold has sneezed repeatedly, touching the same surfaces, etc.). Miguel also knows that HIV is a virus. Using the representativeness heuristic, he groups HIV with other viruses and concludes that, like other viruses, the risk of HIV via casual contact is relatively high.

As in the previous example, Miguel is not making "irrational" decisions. Instead, he is using what he thinks to be true to help him make decisions about probabilities of events that, in his mind, are related. From a scientific standpoint, his inclusion of

HIV with other viruses is wrong in terms of similar modes of transmission. Nonetheless, using the representativeness rule-of-thumb and what he thinks is correct, he groups together similar objects, then makes a decision about risks of HIV transmission. In this case, we could provide useful input to Miguel's decision by giving him correct information about how HIV is transmitted.

There are two aspects of the representativeness heuristic that we want to highlight, both illustrated in the two examples. First, the application of the representativeness rule-of-thumb, like other rules-of-thumb discussed next, may occur almost unconsciously. In all likelihood, if our hypothetical examples came to life, neither Nancy nor Miguel would consciously set out the decision task in the way we described it. Instead, they would move through the steps almost instantaneously. Think about how, earlier, you reacted to the initial description of Steve and the list of professions. Your application of the representativeness heuristic to label him a librarian probably occurred almost instantly. It is doubtful that you carefully considered the details of his description and then self-consciously compared them to your own description of characteristics of farmers, salespeople, airline pilots, librarians, and physicians. This is why we call these *heuristics*, or rules-of-thumb: They are shortcuts to probability decision-making tasks.

Second, it is the *perception* of reality—not the actual reality—that determines how someone will decide on subjective probabilities. If someone is very well informed, his or her perception may match the actual reality. Otherwise, his or her understanding of reality will become the source for decision making. In the example above, Miguel perceived HIV to be like other viruses in the way he understood them to be spread. We know that HIV is not spread through casual contact; that is the reality, based on extensive epidemiological data and theoretical reasoning. For Miguel, however, "reality" for him is that HIV is spread through casual contact. Consequently, he makes decisions that are logical, given this "reality." If we assume he is illogical or stupid, we miss the important point that he, from his viewpoint, is deciding rationally and intelligently. We also miss an important opportunity: understanding how we could change his knowledge—part of his reality—and thus change the conclusions he makes.

Availability   Another important factor in our decision making about probabilities is the availability in memory of items or objects. An item or object that is present in our memory will be judged to be more probable than one that is not present or only weakly so. There are two main contributors to the availability of an item or object in our memory: familiarity and salience.[2] *Familiarity* is the frequency of occurrence of an item or object in our memory, and *salience* is the distinctiveness or vividness of an item or object in our memory, apart from its frequency.

Several examples will help to understand familiarity and salience. The decision-making task is to estimate the percentage of the U.S. population who own cars. This task is given to Paulette, who works and lives in the center of a large U.S. city, and to Tran, who lives and works in a rural area with only a few small towns. Cars are much more familiar in memory to Paulette, who works, lives, and moves around them all day, than they are to Tran, who sees few cars during a day. Because of these differences in familiarity, Paulette will probably overestimate the percentage of the U.S. population with cars and Tran will underestimate it.

Salience is distinct from familiarity. Even if an event or object does not occur frequently, the presence of the event in your mind will be increased if it is dramatic when it does occur. This makes the event more available in memory and thereby increases your perception of its probability. A good example of this is the estimate many people make about the likelihood of an airplane crash: They generally overestimate the likelihood by a wide margin. A primary reason for this is the saliency that an airplane crash has for most people on the rare occasion when it occurs. News pictures of flames leaping from an airplane's wings and windows and of passengers fleeing through smoke and fire make searing images in most people's minds. The saliency of these images makes them available for a long time, increasing personal estimates of the likelihood of occurrence. Contrast this situation with the image most people have of a bicycle crash; namely, no image at all. We would expect people to judge their risk of having a bicycle crash as very remote, given the very low salience of this event and its lack of availability in memory.

The relevance of this factor of availability is easy to see for the case of HIV risk assessments. Those who frequently see or have contact with people with AIDS give higher estimates of the general prevalence of HIV and AIDS, compared with those who have no experience with AIDS or HIV. For example, surveys of citizens in San Francisco, one of the hardest-hit U.S. cities in terms of AIDS, show that they overestimate the prevalence of HIV and AIDS. Images and information about HIV and AIDS are more familiar to them and therefore more available in memory when they are making estimates of HIV infection or AIDS.

An example of the effect of salience is the increase in attention to AIDS that occurs when a well-known figure contracts the disease and the related increase in people's assessments of HIV and AIDS risk. The movie star, Rock Hudson, is credited with bringing the reality of AIDS inadvertently to many Americans for the first time in the mid-1980s. When the news media gave front-page attention to his diagnosis with AIDS and the quick progression of the disease, the salience of AIDS increased sharply for many people. A similar effect occurred when basketball star Magic Johnson revealed that he was HIV positive and was retiring from professional basketball. The news media again gave major coverage to the topic, which increased the saliency of AIDS for many young people, especially African-American youth. In both the Hudson and Johnson cases, health-care workers reported sharp increases in contacts from people who had reassessed and increased their judgment of personal risk for HIV and AIDS. Indeed, in talking about the pattern and frequency of HIV tests, some health-care workers refer to the "Magic Johnson spike"—the greatly increased number of people who sought HIV testing right after Johnson's dramatic announcement.

From our understanding of the factors affecting risk assessments, we can explain these changes in personal risk assessments: major media coverage results in an increase in saliency about AIDS, which, in turn, causes some people to increase their assessment of the presence and risk of HIV and AIDS and of their personal perceived risk of HIV.

Anchoring   The final factor to be covered in explaining the reasons for our subjective probability assessments is anchoring. *Anchoring* is the way in which the starting point for our assessment—that is, our initial estimate or base—affects how we adjust subsequent estimates.

The following example illustrates this factor well.[3] Subjects in a study were asked to estimate the percentage of African countries in the United Nations. They received an arbitrary number between 1 and 100 (by spinning a wheel of fortune), then judged (1) whether the percentage of African countries was higher or lower than this initial number and (2) what the actual percentage was, moving up or down from the initial number. Different groups were, in fact, given different starting points for their estimates, and these seemingly arbitrary initial numbers significantly affected judgments. Groups that received 10 as the initial number gave average estimates of 25 percent for the number of African nations in the United Nations. In sharp contrast, groups that received 65 as the initial number gave average estimates of 45 percent for the number of African nations in the United Nations. These variations occurred even though the subjects understood that the initial numbers were simply random starting points, and the variations persisted even when subjects received payments for accuracy.

For the case of HIV and AIDS risk assessments, the effect of anchoring is demonstrated in the errors people make in assessing the overall risk attributable to a series of events, each with a different probability. As an example, consider this series of possible events: Brad meets Monica, an HIV-infected person; Monica cuts herself on her arm and starts to bleed; Brad has an open cut on his finger; Brad touches Monica's blood with his cut finger. For HIV to be transferred from Monica to Brad, at least these four events would need to occur (and a few other probabilistic events as well, but for the sake of simplicity, we will limit our example to these four events).[4]

Brad's personal risk assessment challenge is to estimate the likelihood of HIV infection from this series of events. If Brad is like most of us, he will overestimate the probability, compared with its actual statistical likelihood. The extent of overestimation can generally be explained by the anchoring heuristic. Brad selects a probability that a new person he meets (Monica) will be HIV-positive, then adds to his probability estimate for each of the other three events occurring. In fact, the overall probability will be smaller than any of the individual events (statisticians can demonstrate this easily). The more events in the series, the lower the probability of the overall conjunctive event occurring. For a conjunctive series of events, then, most lay people, in making their subjective probability assessments, overestimate the overall probability.

There is another main type of risk assessment event series that is relevant to us in considering HIV risk: a disjunctive series. A disjunctive series is one in which A *or* B *or* C *or* D occurs, in contrast to the conjunctive series where A *and* B *and* C *and* D must occur. As an example, consider Christina who had unprotected intercourse with four different men. Her risk assessment challenge is to estimate the HIV risk from all four of these encounters: How likely is it that she contracted HIV from any one of the men? If Christina is like most of us, she will underestimate the actual risk. Christina anchors her subjective probability assessment at a low level for the risk of HIV infection from her first sexual encounter, then makes small adjustments for each of the other three encounters. Typically, these adjustments are not adequate, and the final probability estimate is less than it should be. The probability of a disjunctive series is greater than the probability of each individual event. The more events added to the series, the larger the probability becomes of any one of the events occurring, even if the probability of each individual event is quite small.

These three judgment heuristics—representativeness, availability, and anchoring—help to explain how people handle the difficult task of making subjective probability assessments, of which an HIV risk assessment is a good example. Unfortunately, these judgment shortcuts inadvertently contribute errors that result in risk assessments that are sometimes overestimates and other times underestimates, depending on the judgment task and the heuristic used.

Optimistic Bias

The judgment heuristics we have been discussing are used when we are making subjective probability assessments about risk to others and to ourselves. When we are making these assessments about ourselves, however, another important factor comes into play: optimistic bias. This is also known as personal invulnerability.

Many of us, especially the young, tend to view ourselves as less vulnerable to experiencing bad outcomes. We have an optimistic bias that bad things will not happen to us and, conversely, that good things will happen, compared with other people. This optimistic bias extends into many aspects of our lives, from our wager of several dollars on a lottery ticket to our quick puffs on a cigarette. In the former case, some of us feel that we are luckier than others and therefore that our lottery ticket will be the winning one; in the latter case, some of us feel that our bodies are stronger or healthier than other people's so smoking "just a little" will not do any damage to our lungs and heart. The scientific evidence, however, does not support these personal invulnerability beliefs: The objective chance of winning the lottery is less than the chance of being struck by lightning, and the harmful effects of smoking are cumulative (indeed, non-smokers, who do not even smoke "just a little," suffer damage to their bodies from inhaling smoke from others).

Why do we have this optimistic bias? It arises from our upbringing and is fostered as we grow. Most of us are raised by our families and caregivers to believe that we are special. We are encouraged in this belief as we begin, however tentatively, to deal with the outside world, and we are praised and rewarded for our successes. Our early failures are overlooked and blamed on external circumstances beyond our control. All of this leads us to conclude, usually unconsciously, that good things are associated with us and that bad things are not. The world is just: Good things, we believe, happen to good people and bad things happen to bad people, and we are among the "good people."

This bias toward optimism is beneficial as we grow, because it provides both a reason to continue to attempt activities and a ready explanation for success (namely, that we have the talent or skill) or for failure (namely, that the external circumstances conspired against us this time). In our adolescent years, this bias reaches its peak for many of us, when we see ourselves as invulnerable to many threats and risks. At this extreme point, however, the optimistic bias can blind us to realities, cause us to make incorrect judgments and to take foolhardy actions, and, on occasion, even threaten our life.

In the case of assessing our risk for HIV, the optimistic bias tends to make us underestimate our objective risk for several reasons. First, since the outcomes generally associated with HIV and AIDS are bad, we tend to assume that we are at less risk for bad outcomes than others (research has shown this to be the case for people's judgments about a variety of bad outcomes). Second, we assume the people we are with also are more likely to avoid bad outcomes. These, then, are the "facts" that are in our mind: AIDS, like other bad things, will not happen to me and it will not happen to my friends, lovers, or spouse. Bad things happen to bad people; bad things do not happen to good people, like me and my boyfriend or girlfriend. This perception of the "facts" can lead us to conclude that we are not at risk for HIV from sexual contact with our friends, lovers, and spouse.

The objective facts, however, present a different picture and do not fit neatly into a good person–bad person categorization. Our friends, lovers, and spouses have numerous contacts—some of them sexual—with other people, and we cannot know about all these sexual contacts or about the HIV status of all these other people. Even if we could know all these other people, we would also need to know the HIV status of *all* the other sexual partners of *all* these other people. (There is a further confusing objective fact: the window period associated with the HIV test, which is covered below. For the moment, however, we have more than enough confusing objective facts.) In short, the task of knowing the objective HIV and AIDS risk associated with friends, lovers, and spouses is impossible. Our best choice, therefore, would be to assume the risk of HIV is present and take precautions. The optimistic bias, however, pushes us in the opposite direction: AIDS will not happen to me, especially not from sexual contact with the good people who are my friends and who will not have HIV.

In summary, we see that there are psychological factors that have a major effect on our understanding and interpretation of the "facts" of HIV and AIDS risk. We use judgment heuristics (representativeness, availability, and anchoring) as shortcuts to assess HIV risk for others and ourselves, and these rules-of-thumb are likely to make our subjective probability assessments different from those made by scientists using the objective data. Optimistic bias plays an important role in our personal HIV risk assessments, causing most of us to underestimate our vulnerability to HIV. While there are other factors that can affect risk assessments,[5] the judgment heuristics and the optimistic bias are the important ones for most of us, particularly for our initial assessments.

The most important point about all of these factors is that, in our assessment of our risk for HIV, the objective "facts" are viewed differently by each of us. Our risk assessments are sub-jective—personal evaluations that differ for each of us. Each of us is confronted with a different set of realities in assessing our HIV and AIDS risks, depending on our sexual and drug use behav-iors. When we receive information about HIV and AIDS, we in-terpret this information in the context of our own particular realities. As we interpret the information, we need to be aware of the risk assessment factors that operate to distort our under-standing. We also should be aware of these factors in under-standing why different individuals will come to different assessments of their risk of HIV.

It should now be clear why risk assessment is an uncer-tainty task. It is easy to understand, therefore, why most of us would like a quick and definite answer to the question, "Am I at risk for HIV?" At first thought, the HIV test might seem to be just the method to get this answer. As we discuss next, there is indeed useful information that an HIV test can provide, particularly about the effects of past risks, but it does not provide a guaran-tee of no HIV risk for the present or the future.

HIV TESTING AND RISK ASSESSMENT

Will the HIV test provide the definitive answer to HIV risk? Thuy, for example, might think that both he and his girlfriend, Maricres, should be tested. If they both test HIV negative, he thinks, they can conclude that they are not at risk for HIV and can act on this knowledge. Can the HIV test tell Thuy and Maricres this? To answer this question, we need to review briefly the details of the HIV test.

The Nature and Accuracy of the HIV Test

The biological details of the HIV test are described in Chapter 4. Here, we want to focus on two factors related to the test, which have implications for the information individuals can obtain from the test and the utility of this information in personal risk assessments: the nature of the test and the accuracy of the test.

The Nature of the Test

The HIV tests are antibody tests. As described in Chapter 4, this means that the tests do not directly measure HIV. Instead, they measure whether antibodies to HIV have been produced. As with any virus, there is a time period between infection and the production of antibodies. This is called the *window period*, and, for HIV, this period can be as long as six months. At the beginning of the period, an individual would test HIV negative (seronegative), and, at the end, when antibodies are being produced, the individual is said to have *seroconverted* and would now test HIV positive (seropositive).

These realities of the test mean that a negative HIV test does not necessarily prove that someone is free of HIV; it only proves that the individual did not have antibodies to HIV at the time of the test. Due to the window period, someone can, in fact, have the HIV virus but test HIV negative because no antibodies have been produced yet. This is an important consideration in interpreting test results and drawing conclusions about present and future HIV risk.

There are two other very remote explanations for HIV test results, presented here for the sake of completeness: An individual may test negative and never produce antibodies yet still be infected (due to a quirk in his or her immune system), or an individual may test positive for antibodies but no longer have the virus (due to the lag between the disappearance of a virus and the subsequent disappearance of its associated antibodies from the bloodstream).[6] These two conditions, while possible, are so rare that an individual who has the HIV test and is interpreting the test results need not be concerned with them.

The Accuracy of the Test

The test generally used for HIV antibody testing—the ELISA test—is not 100 percent accurate. Due to the biochemical nature of the test itself and human error in conducting the test, occasional misspecification occurs. As discussed in Chapter 4, there is a very small chance (0.1 percent, less than 1 in 1,000) that the ELISA test will indicate that someone has HIV antibodies when he or she does not (false positive) or that someone does not have HIV antibodies when she or he does (false negative). All positive ELISA tests are checked with another test, the Western blot, to reduce even further the likelihood of a false positive. Consequently, the chance of a false positive test is now extremely small. Negative ELISA tests are not reconfirmed; consequently, the chance of a false negative test remains the same; that is, very small.

With this background, we are in a better position to answer the question, "Will the HIV test provide the definitive answer to HIV risk?" The answer is, "No, not by itself." The accuracy of the test is very high but not perfect. There is the possibility (although very small) of a false negative. The most troublesome aspect, however, is the window period. This problem can be minimized by a retesting, six months after the first. Two HIV negative tests make the possibility of HIV infection unlikely if, in the intervening six months, the individual has not put him- or herself at risk via sex, blood, or birth (see Chapter 7).

For the couple mentioned earlier, Thuy and Maricres, they can be confident that they are HIV negative if they each have two negative HIV tests six months apart and if neither has been exposed to HIV during those six months in the modes applicable to them; namely, sex or blood. Can Thuy and Maricres, therefore, conclude that their personal risk of HIV infection is zero? The answer is, "No."

Risk, as we have seen earlier in this chapter, is always relative. Some people have a very low risk of HIV and others have a high risk. Someone who is not and never has been sexually active may be at no risk for HIV through sexual relations, but this same person could be at risk through accidental contact with infected blood. The HIV test provides valuable information about HIV infection in the past; it does not tell about current or future HIV risk. In reality, we are all at some HIV risk unless we live in a protected cell without any contact with other humans.

The HIV test itself does not tell us if we are at risk for HIV: Only an analysis of modes of HIV transmission and their relationship to our life will give us this information. For many people, the HIV test context provides an excellent opportunity for them to learn about modes of transmission and to consider their relative risks. A very important aspect of this context is the counseling that occurs prior to the test and at the time of the test result.

HIV Test Counseling

Pre-Test and Post-Test Sessions

Taking an HIV test is not like most other tests. The consequences of an HIV test are not the same as, for example, those of an allergy test. A positive HIV test has implications for nearly every aspect of a person's life and raises the likely specter of illness and possibly early death. A negative test, on the other hand, can be misinterpreted as a certification of no HIV risk and, therefore, as a "green light" for behaviors that could put someone at risk of HIV. Both results provide an opportunity for personal risk analysis and the possibility for changes in personal attitudes and behaviors (although, as we will see in the next chapter, the move from knowledge to attitude and behavior changes is not an automatic one).

Because those taking an HIV test may misunderstand the test and its results and because there is an opportunity for education, counseling prior to taking the test and during the explanation of the results has become the accepted procedure. During the pre-test counseling, trained health workers explain what the HIV test does and does not do, what the implications of the different test results are, and what type of reporting and recording will occur (confidential or anonymous). In addition, the counselor explores possible modes of HIV transmission with the individual and assists in personal risk assessment.

The other component of the counseling—the session at which the test results are shared and discussed—is as important as the pre-test counseling. In the not-so-distant past, there were stories of people receiving their test results via mail or even from a message on their home answering machine. In the cases of positive HIV test results, conveying antibody test outcomes in these ways is unethical and cruel, given the implications of a positive result. Even with a negative test result, impersonal communication misses the excellent opportunity to instruct people about HIV and AIDS and about the continuing need to protect themselves. Instead, face-to-face post-test counseling is the standard mode, done by counselors who are prepared to assist people accept and begin to deal with a positive HIV test result or to caution those with a negative test result about such issues as the window period and the need for continuing attention to HIV risk protection.

Recently, home test kits have become available for HIV tests. The controversial aspect of these kits relates to the absence of pre- and post-test counseling. Proponents of wider availability of the home test kits believe that the benefit of having more people tested outweighs the costs of absent or reduced counseling. The counseling itself, some say, is keeping some people from being tested. Opponents of the home test kits argue that many individuals are not equipped to interpret the test result—either positive or negative—correctly. Some individuals, the opponents say, may interpret a negative test result as a certification that they can continue their current behavior, which may involve significant HIV risk to themselves and to others. At this point, the discussion is continuing without resolution.

Confidentiality versus Anonymity of Test Results

There is one other important aspect of the counseling sessions. Is the testing confidential or anonymous?

Confidential testing means that a record of the test result linked to an individual will be maintained, although no information is to exist outside the individual's file. Anonymous testing, however, means that there is no link *ever* between a test result and a person's name. For the purposes of test lab identification, numbers or nonsense names are sometimes attached to HIV test blood and the associated test result. However, only the individual whose blood is being tested knows the number or nonsense name. At many testing sites, those being tested are given one-half of a sheet with the same unique number on both halves. To retrieve the test result, counselors need both halves of the original paper. If someone loses the half-sheet, the results cannot be claimed and the procedure must be started over.

Anonymous testing is superior to confidential testing because there is no way for anonymous test results to be linked to individuals. Because prejudice still exists for those with HIV and AIDS (see Chapter 10), it is better to preclude the possibility of unexpected, unauthorized, or unnecessary disclosure of test results, which can occur under confidential testing conditions but not with anonymous testing. Where there is a choice, therefore, anonymous testing is preferable. When only confidential testing is available, the person being tested should understand the ways that confidentiality will be guaranteed and should feel comfortable with these before proceeding with the test.

At the beginning of this chapter, we presented a model for individual decision making and action involving four steps: knowledge, attitude, intention, and behavior. This chapter has focused on the knowledge and attitude steps with regard to assessments of HIV risk. Based on the outcomes of these assessments, individuals form intentions to take actions—or to take no action—and to maintain or change their behaviors related to HIV risk. As we shall see in the next chapter, knowledge does not automatically result in behavior changes. Preventing HIV transmission and AIDS requires much more than knowledge.

Notes

1. This example, as well as the majority of the judgment heuristics described for the subjective probability model, are drawn from A. Tversky and D. Kahneman, "Judgment Under Uncertainty: Heuristics and Biases," *Science* 185;1974, 1124–1131.

2. The Tversky and Kahneman article (ibid.) discusses other factors contributing to the availability heuristic; familiarity and salience are particularly important ones for our more limited discussion here.

3. Ibid.

4. Two examples of other relevant events: the concentration of HIV in Monica's blood at the time of the bleeding (we know that concentrations vary over time) and the extent to which blood from the cut on Monica's arm has dried by the time Brad touches it (we know that HIV dies quickly when exposed to drying air).

5. These other factors include perceived control over the risk, fear, newness of the risk, and potential for catastrophic outcomes.

6. In the case of an HIV-infected mother, she will pass HIV antibodies to any newborns but may or may not pass HIV. Consequently, her newborn will test HIV positive but may not, in fact, have HIV. It takes up to 18 months for the antibodies to leave the baby's system, in the absence of HIV. If HIV has also been passed, antibodies will continue to be produced and the child will continue to test HIV positive.

Chapter 9

Prevention of AIDS

DISEASE PREVENTION AND HEALTH PROMOTION

MODELS OF HEALTH BEHAVIOR CHANGE

- Health Belief Model
- Health Decision Model
- Precaution-Adoption Process Model

PRINCIPLES OF HEALTH BEHAVIOR CHANGE

- The Cognitive Principle
- The Emotional Principle
- The Behavioral Principle
- The Interpersonal Principle
- The Social Ecological Principle
- The Structural Principle
- The Scientific Principle

EXAMPLES OF HIV AND AIDS PREVENTION PROGRAMS

- AIDS Prevention in Gay and Bisexual Men
- AIDS Prevention among Mexican Migrant Farm Workers

The key to preventing AIDS is to stop the transmission of the HIV virus before it enters the human body. Once inside, the virus cannot be biologically disarmed by a vaccine, based on our current knowledge. (In fact, researchers are not hopeful about the development of an HIV vaccine in the foreseeable future.) Our focus on preventing AIDS, therefore, needs to be on preventing HIV infection. Since we know how HIV is transmitted, we also know how HIV can be blocked from passing from one infected person to another (see Chapter 7). This knowledge needs to be disseminated to anyone who is at risk for HIV and AIDS. In this chapter, we will review general principles of disease prevention, then apply them to the case of AIDS, concluding with two examples of successful AIDS prevention programs.

DISEASE PREVENTION AND HEALTH PROMOTION

The prevention of AIDS would seem to be simple. First, we give the information about stopping HIV transmission to people who are at potential risk, and, second, they act on this information. The information would include suggestions to avoid certain very risky sexual practices, to use condoms, to stop sharing needles, and to avoid direct contact with certain human body fluids (Chapter 7 contains the specific details). Once informed, everyone would follow HIV and AIDS prevention measures and the spread of the virus would be halted, preventing AIDS.

Unfortunately, the task is not at all this simple. Changing HIV and AIDS *knowledge* is different from changing HIV and AIDS *attitudes* and *intentions,* which is different again from changing *behaviors* that could put one at risk for HIV and AIDS. As researchers have discovered with a number of disease prevention practices, people generally are resistant to changing attitudes and behaviors. Why do people not change their health-threatening behaviors when the health risk is obvious and when the means of prevention is clear and effective? Perhaps people do not understand the risk and the way to prevent it. Research has shown, however, that even when people clearly understand a health risk and the means of prevention, they still are resistant to change. Perhaps people do not want to change. Additional research has demonstrated that, even in cases where people understood the risk, accepted the prevention method, and reported that they wanted to and would change, subsequent behavior did not always change.

Health promotion and disease prevention researchers have organized their findings into several models, which highlight important factors explaining why people are resistant to changing their health-related behaviors. In the sections that follow, we turn first to a description of these models and their important concepts and then to a discussion of principles largely derived from these models, which give us guidelines about how to plan and implement effective disease prevention programs. The task is not an easy one, as many have discovered with other disease prevention programs. But, as we will show with several AIDS prevention program examples, when prevention is done well, it can be effective and can change behaviors related to HIV transmission.

MODELS OF HEALTH BEHAVIOR CHANGE

Three models related to health behavior change are particularly useful in understanding HIV and AIDS prevention. These models incorporate concepts and ideas from a long history of research on measuring, establishing, and changing attitudes and behaviors. Each of the three health behavior change models is described below.

Health Belief Model

This model is the oldest of the health behavior change models and grew out of researchers' initial investigations of the reasons for the widespread failure of people to take actions to prevent asymptomatic diseases. (Asymptomatic diseases are those such as lung cancer, where there are no symptoms until the very end of the disease, when death is likely and nothing can be done to reverse the damage. Symptomatic diseases—a cold, for example—have immediate harmful or unpleasant effects that we are aware of; these noticeable effects make it more likely that we will take action.) The health belief model identifies three main variables to explain the absence of action. All three of the variables focus on an individual's perception of different aspects of a health-threatening situation.

The first variable is the person's perceived susceptibility to a health threat. If someone does not see him- or herself as "at risk," this would explain why this person would not change a health-related attitude or practice. In the previous chapter, we discussed the fact that many teenagers do not see themselves at risk for many diseases, including AIDS. Their view of their own susceptibility—their perceived susceptibility—to certain diseases is the critical factor, not the objective measure of their susceptibility. If a person believes that he or she is not susceptible to a disease, no matter what the actual degree of susceptibility may be, that person will not begin the process to take action to protect him- or herself from contracting the disease.

The second important variable is his or her assessment of the severity of the threat. A person may acknowledge that he or she is susceptible to a particular disease but then rate the severity of the threat as too low to worry about. If this person judges the severity to be low, there is not much incentive to take action to protect him- or herself. Again, as was the case with the variable of perceived susceptibility, it is the person's subjective assessment that is important, not the objective measure. We know that AIDS is a deadly disease in almost all cases, a disease with the most severe threat possible. If a person does not know, understand, or accept this, however, that person will continue to underrate the severity of AIDS, and this would be one factor that could explain a lack of action to protect him- or herself.

The third variable is a person's evaluation of the effectiveness of the recommended health-promoting or illness-preventing action. If the action is clearly effective, it is easier for a person to decide to undertake the action or, conversely, it is more difficult for a person to make excuses to avoid taking the action. Seat-belt use in automobiles provides a good example. As the data have become conclusive that seat-belt use saves lives, more drivers have become regular users of seat belts. The HIV and AIDS case provides a different sort of example, one with a more confused outcome. Condoms are promoted as one way to minimize the risk of contracting HIV during sex. Properly used, condoms provide a very large measure of protection but not 100 percent protection. Because condoms are not completely effective, some people have decided that they are not an effective AIDS prevention device. Others, however, see condoms as a generally effective way to prevent the spread of HIV. For those who underrate or denigrate the value of condoms in preventing the spread of AIDS, there is little or no pressure to use them, which could help explain why some people do not use condoms.

Health Decision Model

This model is a more recent reformulation of the Health Belief Model that incorporates variables beyond those related to the individual's views. Decisions about health actions are often made in the context of other people, with other people's views either explicitly considered, in cases where two people must jointly take an action (such as condom use to prevent the spread of HIV), or implicitly considered, in cases where there is an individual action, but it is taken in a social context (such as a decision to stop smoking). The social context is especially important in the case of AIDS. Condom use, for instance, is not only an individual decision but also a decision made by two individuals. When a man and woman decide to use a condom during sex, they make a joint decision, even though it is the man who wears the condom. If the woman favors the use of the condom and the man does not, or vice versa, there is a problem that needs to be jointly resolved.

The Health Decision Model focuses attention on the social variables of experience, knowledge, and interaction, in addition to the three Health Belief Model variables of perceived severity, susceptibility, and evaluation of action. This expanded model acknowledges that decisions to change health-related attitudes and behaviors are made with some attention to our past experiences with other people who are important to us, our knowledge of others' views and opinions, and our current interactions with others.

The Health Decision Model gives us additional insights into why someone might or might not follow a recommended action to prevent the spread of HIV. First, we need to look at the larger social context in which the person lives. For example, in the case of condom use, we need to consider cultural values related to condoms to understand why using condoms might be easy or difficult for people from different cultural groups. In Hispanic culture, for instance, condoms have a number of negative associations (the Catholic Church is against them; prostitutes are associated with them), which would present additional obstacles for a Hispanic male who is considering protection against HIV.

This example can also illustrate the importance of experience and knowledge, the other important social variables in the Health Decision Model. If a Hispanic male has not seen or heard about condoms prior to an AIDS prevention program or has only heard negative things about condoms, it will be even more difficult to convince him to use condoms to prevent HIV infection. He may know about AIDS, see himself as highly susceptible, see AIDS as very serious, and understand that condoms help prevent AIDS, but he still may not take action because of his past knowledge and experience (or lack thereof).

Precaution-Adoption Process Model

Finally, we look at one additional model that has been proposed to help explain why health-related attitudes and behaviors are not easy to change. This mode—the Precaution-Adoption Process Model—focuses on the process of change rather than on particular variables, as the previous two models do. Both the Health Belief Model and the Health Decision Model are static and linear in their view of the health attitude and behavior change process. That is, these models assume that a person moves very logically from A to B to C to D and reaches a decision. For the case of HIV and AIDS risk, for example, a person would assess personal susceptibility to AIDS, severity of the AIDS threat, and the efficacy of the recommended action (say, condom use), using past experience and knowledge, particularly that from discussions and interactions with friends and partners, as important bases to make these assessments. From this assessment, the person makes a decision whether to use a condom.

Laying the situation out in this way highlights how artificial such a process would be for most people. Instead of a smooth, step-by-step decision process, most of us go through a much more complex decision sequence, making one step forward and a half step back, waiting for a while, then taking another step forward, eventually reaching—or backing into—a decision. Some researchers recognized that, for most of us, our decision making is dynamic and fluid, with different factors coming into play in different ways at different times. In the case of AIDS prevention behaviors, for example, certain behaviors (for instance, condom use) require that two people make a joint decision. The important decision factors may be weighed differently for each of them, and, as they move toward a joint decision, the weights of factors may change in different ways, further complicating a final decision and action.

The Precaution-Adoption Process Model proposes that people go through five stages in deciding to make behavior changes. The first stage is awareness or knowledge of a risk or threat. The second stage is acknowledgment of a significant risk to some group of people, while the third stage is acknowledgment of a significant risk to oneself. The fourth stage is deciding to take action to reduce the risk and the fifth stage is actually initiating the behavior. Movement through the stages can be forward or backward as a person's emotions, values, experiences, knowledge, intentions, actions, and social context change over time.

These three models are not in competition with one another but instead are complementary and provide different perspectives on the health attitude and behavior change situation. The more varied our perspectives, the more likely we are to be able to understand obstacles to change and, as important, factors to facilitate change. This is the topic to which we now turn.

PRINCIPLES OF HEALTH BEHAVIOR CHANGE

From the three models just described and from other research as well, researchers and program personnel working in the area of health behavior have developed principles to foster health attitude and behavior change. The set of seven principles,[1] which follows, incorporates factors from the three models and adds several new concepts.

The Cognitive Principle

Correct knowledge must be conveyed to those whom you want to make changes. People need to know the "facts" about HIV, its risks, its spread, and its prevention. Sometimes, this involves conveying new information; other times, it involves correcting misinformation. For the case of AIDS, the cognitive information elements of an AIDS prevention message could include what HIV is, how it is and is not transmitted, how likely people are to become infected, what the consequences of AIDS are, and how AIDS can be prevented.

The cognitive "facts" about HIV and AIDS are numerous (as demonstrated by the length of the earlier chapters in this book). How can we possibly have all the facts in a brief AIDS prevention message? We cannot have and do not need all the AIDS facts in every message. The challenge is to decide which facts are critical to convey and how they can be most effectively conveyed. Generally, this information needs to be simple and in language that is appropriate for the intended target audience. Some of the principles discussed later will help us decide which HIV and AIDS facts need to be conveyed and how these facts can be communicated best. However, HIV and AIDS facts by themselves are necessary but not sufficient for someone to change. We can barrage someone with information, but, unless it is done appropriately, it will not have its intended effect. The other principles discussed here must also be considered in developing an AIDS prevention message.

The Emotional Principle

Change is facilitated when there is a connection to a person's emotions. Rather than simply conveying information to a person, we should have an emotional "hook" with the information. Love or romantic emotions are one choice; think of the number of advertisements that use this emotion for their "hook." Positive emotions generally are better "hooks" than negative emotions, but fear is one emotion that has been effectively used in health behavior change communications. We have to be careful with this particular emotion, however, because, if we generate too much fear, our communication may be missed or may even backfire. An example of this was the early "stop smoking" campaigns, which used such vivid and gory pictures that some smokers literally turned away from the message and never received it, while other smokers either rejected the information outright or decided it was too late to make a change—and kept smoking. To know how much fear is appropriate or to learn which of the other emotions would be best to tap, we need to know and understand well the intended audience for our message. Aspects of several of the other principles presented here can assist in this task.

The Behavioral Principle

We need to recommend specific behaviors, which a person receiving our message should adopt. The more specific the behaviors recommended, the better. For example, a vague communication to "avoid catching AIDS" does not describe the specific behaviors that should be followed. The message, "Use condoms during sex," is much more specific and, therefore, more likely to be followed. However, even this message may not be specific enough for certain target audiences, such as those who have had no experience with condoms. In this case, the message would need to include explicit instructions on how to use a condom, ideally with hands-on experience.

An old AIDS prevention education campaign provides an example of the improper use of this principle. A national advertising firm created an audiovisual AIDS prevention message. The audio portion advised listeners to take precautions to avoid AIDS; the accompanying video component showed a man putting on a sock. The idea was that putting on the sock was to symbolize putting on a condom. Alas, the behavioral message—both audio and video—was too vague to be useful. Indeed, many viewers, not surprisingly, missed the connection between the sock and the condom altogether.

The Interpersonal Principle

An effective message should consider the immediate social network of the target person. Individuals do not exist in isolation; they are part of social groups, both small and large. Because these social groups exert influence on individuals who are part of them, we cannot ignore this influence and still have an effective health behavior change occur. Particularly in the case of AIDS, where the virus is transmitted between individuals, we have to take into account the social network of those we hope to influence with HIV and AIDS protection messages.

Consider the case of a sexually active, heterosexual woman who is our target for a particular AIDS prevention message, namely, to use condoms during sexual relations. Not only must our message convince the woman of the necessity and effectiveness of condom use, but it also must include information about and strategies for negotiating condom use with her male sex partners. We have to convince the woman of the need for protection against AIDS, then train her in ways to convince her sexual partners. This is a very challenging task both for the health promotion campaign and for her. It is a challenging task for the health promotion campaign because each man whom the woman encounters will have a different perspective on the AIDS situation and on the need to use condoms. It is a challenge, therefore, to develop a succinct health promotion message that will address the many different partners the woman may have. The challenge for the woman is even greater. Not only will each potential sexual partner be different in his general attitudes about AIDS and condom use, but each will also vary in his personal mood at the moment when the woman must initiate her AIDS prevention communication.

This example shows how difficult it is to initiate and achieve AIDS prevention measures. We not only have to consider the individual but also the other people who relate to the individual, either on a one-to-one basis (such as the potential sexual partners discussed above) or on a more general basis, such as the members of our family or of a social group, which is particularly important to us. In the cases of our family or our social groups, we need to be aware of the social norms that govern sexual behavior and related AIDS prevention strategies. Consider the case of a homosexual man whose friends do not like to use condoms. We would probably be unsuccessful in our AIDS prevention campaign to him if we focused solely on the risks of HIV and AIDS and why he should use condoms. We would also have to address the social norm operating in his group of friends that condom use is viewed negatively. We would first have to know more about why his friends have this negative view (the feel of sex using a condom? the inconvenience of using a condom? the associations with using a condom; such as, it could imply that someone does not trust his partner?) and then develop our message to address the specific concerns.

The Social Ecological Principle

General social and cultural issues specifically relevant to the target individuals should be considered in developing effective HIV prevention programs. The Interpersonal Principle recognizes the importance of those people who surround the target individual in achieving change in health attitudes and behaviors. We could consider this the inner circle of social influence. The Social Ecological Principle recognizes the importance of circles of individuals beyond this inner circle and the interrelatedness of all these circles of social influence that radiate out from our target individual. In particular, the Social Ecological Principle addresses the importance of the social and cultural dimensions.

All of us are part of different social and cultural groups. These groups have norms—or standards of behavior—about many activities, including sexual activity and drug use, the two behaviors in which we are most interested as AIDS prevention specialists. To be effective AIDS educators, we must be aware of the particular social and cultural norms related to AIDS of the groups to which our target individual belongs and of how these norms are similar to or in conflict with AIDS prevention guidelines. In addition, the AIDS educator should recognize the benefits—and sometimes the necessity—of establishing new social norms that promote AIDS prevention. When the social "atmosphere" promotes change toward AIDS prevention, rather than discouraging it, it becomes easier for the individual to initiate and follow through on AIDS-preventing activities.

The situation with AIDS education and drug users presents a good example of the need to attend to social and cultural norms. If we consider only the Cognitive Principle in developing an AIDS prevention message related to drug use, the message is straightforward: Use new needles for IV drugs, do not share needles, and clean needles with bleach if you must share them. In the United States, this message has generated controversy, not because the facts are wrong but because the content clashes with general social norms. The drug user or those in his or her inner circle may accept the content of the message, but others in the outer circles of the general population resist the message because they disagree with any recognition that someone is using drugs. For example, some of those in the outer circle say that providing people with clean needles or telling people to clean their used needles legitimizes drug use. They prefer the message "don't use drugs." Unfortunately for the drug user, it is not a simple matter of stopping drug use; there is a physical addiction that cannot be easily satisfied. In addition, the drug user is part of a subculture where drug use is accepted and the social norm is to continue the behavior.

The approach that AIDS educators have generally taken to solve this conflict is to develop programs for particular groups of drug users, using their social norms as the basis and starting point for AIDS prevention actions. Since the general population is not the target population, AIDS educators working with drug users usually keep a low profile in the general community so as to minimize the conflict with social norms that do not admit to or recognize the realities of drug use.

The Social Ecological Principle also directs our attention to the necessity of having role models or leaders who are part of the health campaign. Our message can be much more effective coming from a respected leader than from an unknown announcer. If the model or leader is viewed as a social norm setter, his or her message will have more effect on the appropriate listener because there is a bridge between the individual's inner and outer circles of social influence. The challenge is to pick the most appropriate role model for the particular individuals whom we want to affect. We will need different models for different individuals and even different models for the same individuals as the situation changes. For instance, we may need one type of role model when we are first convincing someone to use condoms, then a different type of model when we are providing more detailed instruction about the use of condoms, about how to negotiate condom use with a sexual partner, or about maintaining condom use over time.

The Structural Principle

An effective prevention program considers the laws, technology, and physical settings relevant to the target individuals. The context in which an individual lives involves not only social and cultural dimensions, as we have discussed above, but also laws, technology, and physical settings. These latter aspects are considered the structural elements and they can complement or conflict with the social and cultural norms. For instance, laws are the codification of some social and cultural norms, but frequently there is a gap between current laws and current norms, especially on sensitive social issues like AIDS. The AIDS prevention specialist, therefore, must be aware of these realities too when he or she develops an AIDS prevention campaign. In important ways, the structural elements can support or hinder health promotion messages and programs.

A good example of the power of structural elements in health promotion campaigns is provided by the case of efforts to decrease smoking. The data (that is, the cognitive aspects) are clear on the harmful effects of smoking on the smoker and on those in his or her environment. Smokers generally were aware of these deleterious effects, but this knowledge alone was not usually sufficient for them to stop smoking. In addition, certain groups (especially young women) were continuing to smoke. Following the lackluster success of antismoking campaigns aimed at the general population, antismoking advocates changed their strategy to focus on structural changes. Now, there are laws regulating smoking and physical barriers to smoking, such as the nonsmoking rule on all U.S. domestic airlines and the increasing number of nonsmoking rules for restaurants and other public places.

In the case of AIDS, structural elements are equally useful. For example, we encourage people who are at high risk for AIDS to be tested for HIV. Before we promote this activity, however, we have to have enough testing sites in place with enough well-trained counselors to carry through on the benefits of testing. Likewise, laws have to be in place providing for anonymous testing, in the ideal case, or confidential testing, at a minimum, to eliminate or minimize potential harmful consequences of the release of results.

Another good example of the importance of structural elements relates to the issue of condoms. Condoms are widely advocated as good protection against HIV transmission. Because condoms are not 100 percent protection, it has been important to increase the quality of condoms. Now, tests are routinely conducted on the structural integrity of condoms, and the results are disseminated to increase the availability of the highest quality condoms. Because high-quality condoms are a necessary, although not a sufficient, condition for preventing HIV transmission during sexual intercourse, this attention to the structural aspect has been important.

There has been a different sort of attention to other physical aspects of condoms. Condoms now are available in a variety of styles, sizes, and colors to increase their attractiveness to potential users. A female condom (that is, a plastic sack-like device inserted into the vagina) has also been developed, although its effectiveness is still being tested. There are stores in some major

U.S. cities devoted largely to condoms. (Interestingly and importantly, these stores also create a social setting—think back to the Social Ecological Principle—in which condoms are the norm and the focus of attention; this helps to reorient social norms surrounding condoms, changing them from a taboo topic to a common—even humorous—topic.)

The Scientific Principle

Scientific methods must be used to research the target audience while developing an HIV and AIDS prevention program, then to assess the effectiveness of the program that is created. Our AIDS prevention materials and campaigns must be subjected to the ultimate scientific test: In practice, are the materials effective? Scientific research methods can help us determine deficits in AIDS knowledge or current AIDS-related social norms for a particular target group. This information will help create programs likely to be effective, but it is not sufficient to develop and implement an AIDS prevention program. Using scientific methods, the health promotion specialist must test the effectiveness of the program to be sure that it was implemented as planned and to determine its positive and negative consequences.

The best way to determine these issues is to conduct a scientific evaluation of every AIDS prevention program. In a typical scientific evaluation, quantitative indices of the program's goals are developed. Two identical groups are formed from members of the target audience. Baseline measures are made on members of the groups before the program begins. Then, one of the groups receives the program and the other, serving as the control, does not. (On occasion, the control group receives a limited version of the program or a different program.) After the program is concluded, both groups are measured again to detect changes due to the AIDS prevention program. In addition to quantitative measures, interviews are frequently conducted with those in the program to obtain information about their experiences—both positive and negative—with the program components. Sometimes, we inadvertently cause some changes—sometimes for the better and sometimes for the worse—when we implement a health promotion program and only the participants can tell us about these.

Increasingly, program evaluation is becoming a regular part of AIDS prevention programs. At the outset of the AIDS crisis, there was a tendency to rush to implement any type of program, without sufficient attention to its consequences. The lack of changes from some of the early AIDS education campaigns caused those involved in AIDS prevention to take a harder look at the concrete results of their efforts. The two examples that follow provide good examples of how AIDS education programs can be evaluated.

EXAMPLES OF HIV AND AIDS PREVENTION PROGRAMS

The two AIDS prevention programs described below incorporate aspects of many of the seven principles of health behavior change. The two programs are very different: The first program focuses on homosexual and bisexual men and the second on Mexican migrant farm workers.

AIDS Prevention in Gay and Bisexual Men[2]

This program was conducted in the Pittsburgh area in 1986 and 1987. It involved nearly 600 gay and bisexual men who volunteered to be in an AIDS prevention program. The program had two components, the first of which was an hour-long small-group lecture, led by a gay health educator, about AIDS and its consequences and how to prevent the transmission of HIV (focusing on condom use during anal sex). About half of the men, determined on a random basis, participated in only this component.

From our analysis of health behavior change principles earlier in this chapter, we see that this first program component (the small-group lecture) is based largely on the Cognitive Principle. That is, men were given the facts about HIV and AIDS and were encouraged to make changes. The use of a gay health educator also incorporates some aspects of the Interpersonal Principle, in that the participants had one-to-one contact with a professional man similar to them, thereby making it easier for the participants to identify with the speaker and accept what he was saying about condom use.

The other group of men in the program participated in the first component (small-group lecture) but also in another: skills training. During the second program component, which lasted about a hour, the men learned the skill of condom negotiation and generated among themselves new norms about "safer" sex. This second component was led by a psychotherapist from a community organization that provided counseling services to sexual minorities, such as gay and bisexual men. The second component involved role playing between the men and discussion among them about safer sex and sexuality.

We can see that the second program component incorporated the Emotional Principle (in the role playing situations); the Behavioral Principle (in the skill training, which occurred related to negotiating condom use with a sexual partner); the Interpersonal Principle (in the friendly relationships that were developed among the men during the course of their discussions); and the Social Ecological Principle (in the new social norm setting that occurred among the men during their discussions).

The Scientific Principle was central to this program. All the men were given questionnaires about their AIDS-related knowledge and behaviors before the program began and after the program was over (we will concentrate here on the first follow-up six months later). The test group was the "small-group lecture plus skills training" group; the control group was the "small-group lecture" group. The main focus of the research was the effectiveness of the skills training.

The scientific study results indicated that men in both the control group and the test group had similarly high levels of knowledge before the program began and this level stayed high in the postprogram assessments. The small-group lecture component, therefore, did not make much change in HIV and AIDS knowledge because there was little change that needed to be made: Most of the men already knew all the facts about AIDS and its prevention.

The small-group lecture plus skills training component, however, had the promise of affecting other areas, beyond knowledge. Did it do so? We are able to answer this question because the men in the small-group lecture component served as the comparison base (control group) against which to judge changes in the men in the test group (small-group lecture plus skills training).

The target behavior advocated by the program was condom use during anal sex with a man. Among other questions, the researchers asked how many times the men had used condoms during insertive anal intercourse during the past six months. By following the answers to this question over time, the researchers were able to see the effects of the AIDS prevention program. The men in the control group showed no before-after change in this target behavior: The men reported using condoms with about 40 percent of their partners and this percentage did not change after they received the small-group lecture. This, then, was the basis against which to judge the test group, who received both the small-group lecture and the skills training. These men, as we would expect, started at about the same level before the program: They too reported using condoms with about 40 percent of their sexual partners. But after the program, they reported a significant change: They had used condoms for insertive anal intercourse with about 70 percent of their partners.

The small-group lecture plus skills training was probably effective because it incorporated more aspects related to more health behavior change principles and, in particular, focused on areas where the men were in need of assistance: behavioral skills training and norm resetting related to sexual practices. This component, therefore, had the potential to have a bigger effect and the results demonstrated that it did.

AIDS Prevention among Mexican Migrant Farm Workers[3]

This program was conducted in Southern California in 1991. It involved about 300 male farm workers who traveled to the United States to pick crops in the agriculture fields. Migrant workers in this area are at risk for AIDS because prostitutes are regularly brought through the camps where they live. These prostitutes are themselves sometimes infected with HIV and, due to the large number and rapidity of sexual contacts these women have with farm workers, there is the risk for the spread of HIV. A program was developed to instruct the farm workers about AIDS and about the need to use condoms with prostitutes.

The main component of the program was a *fotonovela*—an eight-page photo storybook with pictures and captions. Figure 9–1 provides a sample of some of the fotonovela panels. The story tells of three farm workers who work in the fields, meet prostitutes, and, through the prostitutes, learn about the need to use condoms. In addition, condoms were provided, as were instructions on how to use them. (The program had other components, but we will not focus on those aspects here.) The program was developed with farm worker input about the best approach to take with such culturally sensitive issues as condoms. Farm workers also served as models for the photos.

The scientific study involved using small groups of farm workers, all of whom were tested about AIDS-related knowledge, attitudes, and behaviors—the before (baseline) measure. Then, about two-thirds of the men (the test group) received the materials, while the other men did not and served as a control to assess the effects of the materials over about a month's time. Then, all the men were again tested—the after measure—and the fotonovela was given to the one-third of the men who had not yet received it.

In terms of the health behavior change principles, we can see that several principles are involved in this intervention: the Cognitive, Behavioral, Social Ecological, Structural, and Scientific Principles; the Emotional Principle was also included in the content of the story. The knowledge and facts about AIDS conveyed by the fotonovela involve the Cognitive Principle. The explicit instruction about how to use a condom relates to the Behavioral Principle. The Social Ecological Principle is involved in the use of farm worker and prostitute models in the photos with which the men could identify. (Preliminary research, for instance, showed that the prostitute who advocated condom use was viewed by the men as a "higher class" prostitute, exactly the type, they said, who would believably advocate condom use.) The Social Ecological Principle was also involved in the social and cultural considerations taken into account for the format of the AIDS materials; a fotonovela is a format with which the men are very familiar in Mexico and one that is at an appropriate literacy level. The Structural Principle was also involved: The condoms given to the men were specially selected not only for high quality but also for a degree of lubrication that these men

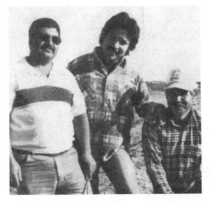

Marco, Sergio and Victor—three men who leave their town in search of opportunities, they confront danger!

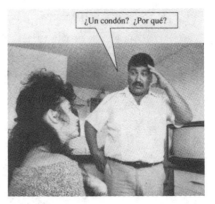

A condom? Why?

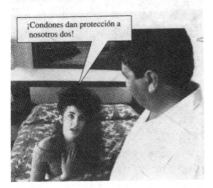

Condoms give protection to both of us!

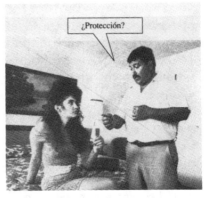

Protection?

Figure 9–1

Sample Set of Photos from the Fotonovela, "Tres Hombres Sin Fronteras" (Three Men Without Borders), an AIDS Prevention Photo Booklet for Mexican Migrant Farm Workers[4]

were known to prefer. Finally, the Scientific Principle was involved in the development of the materials and in the design of the study assessing the effects of the materials.

In brief, the results showed that all of these men knew many of the facts about AIDS even before participating in the program. The fotonovela materials resulted in small but significant changes in knowledge (comparing the "before" and "after"

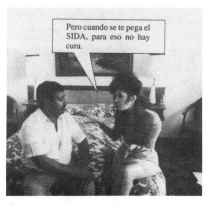

Yes, protection against diseases like gonorrhea, syphilis, even AIDS!

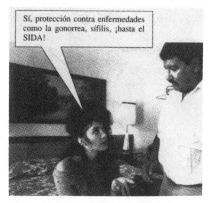

Because when you get AIDS, there isn't a cure for that.

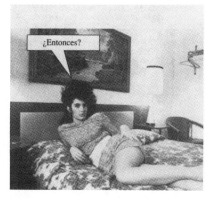

So then?

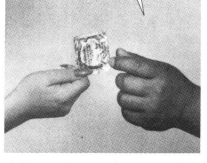

OK!

measures of the men in the test and control groups). The most significant changes were in reported condom use with a prostitute—the target behavior. Among the men who had received the fotonovela and who had the opportunity to use a condom with a prostitute, all but one had used condoms. Among the control group of men who had not received the fotonovela and who had the opportunity to use a condom with a prostitute, none had used a condom. The behavior changes seemed to occur with men for whom the fotonovela materials were particularly well suited in terms of their cultural and social norms. One lesson is that AIDS prevention materials must be very carefully targeted, taking into consideration all of the principles we have reviewed.

While both of these AIDS prevention programs produced positive changes, neither caused perfect compliance with AIDS prevention methods. In the gay and bisexual men study, some of the men were still engaging in risky sexual behaviors. In the migrant worker study, men at one of the camps did not make the desired behavior changes. These less-than-perfect outcomes remind us that the path from new health-related knowledge to changes in attitudes, intentions, and behaviors is a challenging one. With the help of the Scientific Principle, we can identify when and why we are successful and build on these factors, and we can identify when and why we are not successful, then change these factors to make the program better.

In this chapter, we have focused on the challenge of preventing HIV transmission and AIDS. As the two examples showed, successful AIDS prevention involves careful attention to the cognitive, emotional, behavioral, interpersonal, and social ecological situation of the targeted individuals, as well as attention to the structural aspects of the context in which the targeted individuals live. Once we have considered all of these aspects, we are then ready to develop our AIDS prevention program. When we implement the program, we need to carefully assess its effectiveness, with a rigorous scientific approach. Our scientific assessment must be a regular part of the program because people and situations change and we need to be aware of those changes.

Notes

1. This set is an expansion of a related formulation in L. Liskin, C.A. Church, P. T. Piotrow, and J. A. Harris, "AIDS Education: A Beginning," *Population Reports*, September 1989, (Series L); 8.

2. Full details are in R. O. Valdiserri, D. W. Lyter, L. C. Leviton, C. M. Callahan, L. A. Kingsley, and C. R. Rinaldo, "Variables Influencing Condom Use in a Cohort of Gay and Bisexual Men," *Am. J. Public Health 78*; 1989: 801–805.

3. More details are in R. Conner, "Preventing AIDS among Migrant Latino Workers: An Intervention and Model," *Wellness Lecture Series*. Oakland, Calif.: University of California/Health Net, 1992.

4. These materials were developed by the Novela Health Foundation, supported by a grant from the California Community Foundation; used with permission. The study of the materials' effectiveness was also supported in part by the California Community Foundation, along with the support of the American Foundation for AIDS Research.

Chapter 10

Living with AIDS: Human and Societal Dimensions

THEORETICAL PERSPECTIVES FROM SOCIAL PSYCHOLOGY

- Role Theories
- Cognitive Theories

HUMAN DIMENSIONS OF HIV AND AIDS

- Confronting the News of Infection
- Accepting the Reality of Infection

SOCIETAL DIMENSIONS OF HIV AND AIDS

- Prejudice
- Discrimination

All of us are living with AIDS. Some of us have HIV, others have full-blown AIDS, and others are HIV negative. Nonetheless, all of us, as members of our society, are living with the realities of HIV and AIDS, either indirectly or directly.

We frequently hear about "PWAs," people living with AIDS. These are HIV-positive people directly living with AIDS day in and day out. There are others living with AIDS almost as directly because their spouse, lover, brother or sister, roommate, or neighbor is HIV positive. The rest are living more indirectly with AIDS. This may involve knowing that others in our community are infected with HIV, or it may involve other, more distanced aspects (such as effects of HIV infection on our health-care system or on our social service network).

Everyone in our society, therefore, and, increasingly, in every society around the world, lives with HIV and AIDS. In this chapter, we will analyze two aspects of living with AIDS: the human dimension and the societal dimension. The section on the human dimension will focus primarily on those who are HIV positive and the challenges they face. The section on the societal dimension will focus on some important aspects of society's reaction to those with HIV and AIDS and the reasons for these reactions. In this chapter, we draw on research from the field of social psychology, which studies the reasons for and effects of human interactions of all types. As the basis for our discussion of the human and societal dimensions of HIV and AIDS, therefore, we need first to understand two important sets of theoretical perspectives from social psychology.

THEORETICAL PERSPECTIVES FROM SOCIAL PSYCHOLOGY

The field of social psychology concentrates on human behavior in groups. Many aspects of our behavior are determined by the direct or indirect influences of others, even some aspects that we may think of as "innate" or "inside" of us and, therefore, beyond the control of others. For example, our self-concept is formed and reformed in interaction with others. Our attitudes and beliefs also are shaped and reshaped through discussion and interchange with other people. Indeed, because we are social animals who live in groups, there are few aspects of our inner or outer selves that are not affected by other people.

Social psychologists over the past century have developed theories to explain different aspects of people's behaviors in groups. No theory explains all aspects of people's behaviors, but theories taking a similar approach have been useful in explaining different parts of people's behaviors. These similar approaches can be grouped into three general theoretical perspectives.[1] These three perspectives are role theories, learning theories, and cognitive theories. Role theories and cognitive theories are particularly relevant to our understanding of the human and societal dimensions of HIV and AIDS. Consequently, these perspectives will be described in more detail below. For the sake of completeness, learning theories can be briefly described here as those that focus on the relationship between stimuli (such as rewards and punishments) and responses (such as changes in personal behavior). From this perspective, for example, human behavior is viewed as being affected by an exchange of rewards (both concrete ones like money and abstract ones like prestige). While there are aspects of the human and societal dimensions of AIDS that are illuminated by this theoretical perspective, it is less relevant to us than are the other two theoretical perspectives from social psychology, to which we now turn.

Role Theories

The basic idea that underlies this set of theoretical perspectives is that the roles we have are significant determinants of the ways we interact with others and the ways others interact with us. Before we progress further, we should raise a caution: The theatrical concept of a "role" being played on stage is not the correct conception of "role" for this set of theories. A theatrical role is one that is superficially adopted by the actor, not a role that "gets below the skin." Also, the theatrical idea of role has the connotation of artificiality; an actor can decide to "play" a role and behave in artificial ways dictated by the role.

In contrast, role theorists see roles as the fibers of the social network that interlinks all of us. Think of the unit of analysis—the focus point—as the social group, not the individual. From a social group perspective, roles link people, in particular through expectations about and understandings of roles. These understandings and expectations are the main motivators of and explanations for behaviors.

To understand this theoretical perspective better, think of just one of the roles that many readers may have: the role of student. (All of us have multiple roles, so, for a complete picture, we would need to analyze all the person's roles. For the moment, however, we will focus on just a single role.) As a student, you understand that you have certain obligations and responsibilities, such as attending class, doing reading, asking questions, writing papers, and taking examinations. In return, others in related roles, in particular your instructor or professor, also have obligations and responsibilities related to your role, such as assigning readings, giving lectures, passing on information and ideas, reviewing your written work, grading your exams, and providing grades. These role expectations are very real and order the interactions of students and professors.

To understand just how real these expectations are, think of cases where some of the role expectations are not being met. Imagine an instance where the professor never attends class, never lectures, and never answers questions. You, in your student role, are justifiably upset when this occurs because this social interaction is not a balanced one: The professor will still assign a grade. One way to resolve the issue would be to drop the class and thus end the role interconnection. (Note in this example that the upset that the student experiences does not relate to anything "on the inside" of either the student or the professor, such as personality issues; instead, it is the result of mismatched role expectations.)

Role expectations are also known as *norms*—socially defined standards of behavior that guide individual actions. In the example above about the student and professor, the sample obligations and responsibilities (for example, taking tests) are norms that relate to the acceptable performance of these roles. Without norms, we would not know what should properly occur between a student and a professor, and people in these roles would not know how they were expected to behave. Some roles have very clear norms on which everyone in a social group agrees (for example, the role of driver of an automobile) and others (for example, citizen of the world) have poorly defined norms about which different people may disagree.

In Chapter 9, we first discussed norms as one factor that can affect people's decisions to protect themselves from HIV infection. In the social interaction involving the roles of lovers, there are norms about behaviors that are part of these roles (such as having sexual encounters) and, for some people, norms about using protection (such as condoms) during these encounters. HIV and AIDS prevention programs, like those we described at the end of the last chapter, can have as one of their aims to make particular norms more conscious for people and also more definitive (that is, condoms must be used for vaginal and anal sexual intercourse.)

Role theories will be useful to us later in this chapter when we consider such human issues as role conflicts for PWAs or between PWAs and others with whom they interact. These types of theories will also help to explain such societal issues as prejudice and discrimination against those with HIV and AIDS.

Cognitive Theories

The other set of theoretical perspectives we will discuss are very different from the role theories. In contrast to role theories, cognitive theories focus on the conceptions inside people's minds, not factors (such as roles) in the outside world. The basic idea behind cognitive theories is that mental conceptions (also known as *cognitions*) give us a framework both for interpreting experiences and for shaping our actions. Cognitions are mental representations of knowledge or thoughts, not feelings or actions. Related individual cognitions are combined in our minds into cognitive structures, known as *schemas.* These schemas serve as reference points for organizing past experiences or interpreting new experiences, or they serve as templates for activating new ideas. These mental representations undergo mental processing that eventually leads to action or inaction. While our minds process schemas of all types and on all subjects, we are most concerned here with social cognitions, those cognitions focused on people in our lives and our interactions with them.

An example will help to illustrate the perspective and utility of cognitive theories, with particular attention to social cognition. Vivian and her friend Joy see a poster describing a panel discussion by PWAs that is to occur later in the week. Assume that Vivian has taken a class on HIV and AIDS and, therefore, has some experiences and knowledge related to AIDS. Joy, however, has not taken an AIDS class and has never seen anyone with AIDS except for an occasional news report on TV. What do Vivian and Joy think when they see the poster about the PWA panel? Each of them will unconsciously draw on the schemas in her mind to envision what the PWA panel might entail and, based on this, to decide whether to take action. It is important to remember that the mental processes we will describe below happen almost instantaneously. To understand where these processes come from and how they operate, however, we need to slow down the mental process. Consequently, in the descriptions below, the mental processing steps are set out in sequential fashion and with a self-consciousness that is not typical of their normal, instantaneous operation.

Let's consider the cognitive processes for Vivian first. Vivian has studied HIV and AIDS, has seen videotapes in class about PWAs, and has met several PWAs. All of these experiences have resulted in cognitions for Vivian; these cognitions will have been stored in her mind and united into a schema about PWAs. When Vivian sees the poster about the panel, this schema is activated, along with other related schema (for example, her schema about a panel). These schemas will make Vivian think of a small group of people who reflect the HIV situation as she understands it in her community: somewhat more men than women, somewhat younger than a random group of people, perhaps one drug user, and probably several people of minority racial/ethnic status. Otherwise, Vivian pictures a panel that looks like most any other panel. She also imagines that the panel members will behave like most other panels, with the notable exceptions that they will be more personally revealing and candid and they will discuss matters that are not usually part of most panels (sexual behavior, family reactions, finances, etc.).

Joy has a much different picture in her mind when she reads the poster. Because she has had no direct knowledge about HIV and AIDS and no experience with anyone who is HIV positive, she does not have the well-developed schemas upon which Vivian can draw to interpret the poster. Instead, Joy draws on (almost unconsciously and instantaneously, remember) schemas about a panel and about HIV and AIDS based on a few television camera shots. Joy pictures a group of very sick people, some coughing, some in wheelchairs, one very angry and belligerent.

Who do you think is more likely to attend the PWA panel? Vivian is probably your choice. Why? She has a clearer idea about who and what the panel will involve, and these cognitions have positive or neutral connotations. For Joy, the cognitions are vague and they have negative connotations (sickness, anger, bitterness). Unless other positive cognitions are activated for Joy (perhaps the opportunity to have dinner before the panel with her friend Vivian), it is unlikely Joy will attend the panel.

Note how, in this example, cognitions and schemas are brought instantly into play in interpreting new reality. Then, from this interpretation, the likelihood of experiencing the event begins to vary. Joy would probably benefit more from attending the PWA panel than Vivian, since the experience would be a very new and different one for her. (She would be struck, for instance, by the normalcy of the look of the panel.) But, because of the way cognitive processes work, Joy is unlikely to attend. Even if her friend Vivian tries to convince her to attend, the images in Joy's mind are difficult barriers to overcome. Remember, too, that these images may be just outside of consciousness to Joy and, to the extent she is aware of them, she may be reluctant to share them with Vivian. It is easier for her to tell Vivian, "I'd love to go, but I'm busy that evening."

Before we leave cognitive theories, there are a few additional concepts to discuss. First, social cognitions are unique in that the objects on which they are based—people—have a tendency to change and add a new external reality with which our minds need to deal. If our friend Duane, for example, changes jobs or changes wives or even changes haircuts, our mentally stored schema related to him will be somewhat at odds with the new reality he presents. The stored schema will need some adjustments, but these adjustments are made against the background of the old schema, which exerts a conservative, status-quo pressure. Every time a schema is activated, it undergoes some adjustments and expansion, and is then restored in a strengthened form. Frequently activated schemas, such as those related to our own self-concept, are well established in our cognitive structures and become better established—and, therefore, more difficult to change—with each new activation.

Second, our cognitions—and especially our social cognitions—form a generally balanced and ordered whole. Think again to the example of changes in our friend Duane. While our schema of Duane may have both positive and negative components, these cognitive components are balanced to create a schema that has an internal consistency. Imagine that we learn from a friend that Duane has been arrested for bank robbery. This news, completely contradictory to any of our schema components, presents a *cognitive dissonance*—an imbalance in our cognitive conceptions—that needs resolution. Our first reaction might be that Duane was mistaken for someone else, which would resolve the cognitive dissonance. Another reaction could be that Duane was at the wrong place at the wrong time: He was at the bank to make a deposit but was kidnapped under pressure and forced by others to be the front man in the robbery. Either of these explanations brings our old schema of Duane (as a law-abiding person) into line with the new reality and puts the schema back into balance.

Cognitive theories will be useful to us in this chapter when we consider such human issues as self-esteem and self-concept for PWAs or those interacting with them. The cognitive perspective will also help to explain such societal issues as stereotyping those with HIV and AIDS and the difficulty of changing people's attitudes and opinions. We had a preview of some of these issues in Chapter 9, in our discussion of the difficulties of getting people to change well-established attitudes, beliefs, and behaviors that put them at risk for HIV infection.

With these two theoretical perspectives as background, we now are ready to explore and better understand some of the human and societal dimensions to living with AIDS.

HUMAN DIMENSIONS OF HIV AND AIDS

Those living most directly with HIV and AIDS are people infected with the virus. These individuals have significant challenges—psychological, social, and physical—in dealing with HIV. They also have significant opportunities not open to the rest of us. In this section, we will explore these challenges and opportunities, using perspectives from both role theory and cognitive theory.

Confronting the News of Infection

Many HIV-positive people first learn about their seropositive status when they have an HIV test. Others receive this news when they develop their first opportunistic infection and, in the course of working with their doctor to diagnose this physiological change, learn that they are HIV positive. In both cases, although the mental processes can vary, it can be a significant challenge to deal with the new information concerning HIV infection. In each case, however, the news of HIV infection puts major pressure on the individual's self-concept.

Self-Concept

The self is probably one of the most developed schemas each of us has in our mind. Although we may not often be aware of the fact, our self is a social construct, developed and maintained in interaction with others. If those around us make sudden changes in their behavior toward us, we quickly become conscious of the importance of others' appraisals in how we view ourselves. Usually, however, changes in others' behaviors toward us are subtle and do not occur all at once. Consequently, only minor adjustments are usually made in our self-concept.

As we discussed in the section on the cognitive perspective, schemas are reinforced each time they are activated. The self-schema, since it is regularly activated, is one of the strongest schemas in most people's cognitive structure. Parts of the self-schema can vary and minor adjustments are regularly made, but, by and large, we have a constant and firm self-concept. One part of the self-schema that varies is our self-esteem, our positive or negative evaluation of ourselves. A series of good experiences can boost our self-esteem and a series of bad ones can dampen our self-esteem. Nonetheless, most people have a fairly constant appraisal of themselves, built up through experiences that anchor their self-esteem at a high or low level.

Consider, then, the cognitive situation Fernando confronts when he learns he is HIV positive. This news is a direct and significant threat to his self-concept. Making matters more difficult is the fact that Fernando does not seem any different than he was prior to the news of the test: He is still healthy and confident, a good swimmer, a bad singer, a good son, a thoughtful friend, etc. But, out of the blue, he receives news that puts all of this in jeopardy.

It is understandable, from a cognitive perspective, that Fernando's first reaction would be denial. This new piece of information does not fit into his self-concept. Indeed, to accommodate the reality of HIV-positive status, Fernando will have to change many aspects of his self-concept—something that none of us does quickly or easily. Moreover, other than the HIV test counselor who does not play a large role in Fernando's life, there is no one else who knows this information. Fernando may simply decide that the test result is wrong, thereby denying the new information and preserving his self-concept. Good HIV test counselors are prepared for this reaction and realize the tremendous pressure that exists in all of us to maintain our current self-concept. The HIV test counselor may encourage Fernando to have a second HIV test, not because she thinks the test result is wrong (although there is a very, very small chance of this; see Chapter 8) but instead because it will give Fernando time to think about the new information and add another piece of information supporting the first.

One reaction the counselor wants to avoid is forcing Fernando to fit this new information into his self-concept. It may cause him to turn against the news in understandable but dangerous ways. For instance, Fernando could set out to reinforce his current self-concept (that he is HIV negative) by engaging in risky sexual behaviors, which, to him, "proves" that he is not HIV positive and, at the same time, reinforces his concept of himself as a sexually desirable man. Other troubling cognitions (for example, that he is socially and morally irresponsible to put others at risk for HIV) may, for the time being, be avoided.

While many people who learn they are HIV positive (without any other outward signs of AIDS) may go through a period of denial, most do not act out their anger at the news in this way. Instead, they do what most of us do when a very serious threat to our self-concept arises: They talk to their closest, most important friends. Since we define ourselves through our interaction with others, we also redefine ourselves this way. This is not an easy step, however, because we are not sure how our friends will react. Will they think we are diseased and never see us again? Will they still love us, even though they do not fully understand HIV and AIDS? Will they still have sexual relations with us if we use protections (such as condoms)? These questions raise issues of role experiences and expectations, which can be understood more completely if we shift to the role theory perspective.

Role Experiences and Expectations

As discussed in the sections above, we interact with others in terms of roles which are more or less well defined. Among people with whom we interact regularly, these roles are well defined, although they usually are not explicitly articulated. Instead, the dimensions of the roles are created in interaction over a long period of time and adjustments are made as the individuals change and grow. Sometimes, these adjustments make the roles more formal and distance the individuals; other times, the adjustments open up new dimensions to the roles and increase the closeness between the people.

The individual dealing with the news of HIV infection commonly will turn to good friends and family. Just as this news is threatening to his or her self-concept, the new information about HIV infection can be threatening to the role expectations that good friends and family share. Frequently, this one piece of news raises other issues that also may be new. The more issues raised, the more potentially threatening the news can be to the role experiences and expectations of a well-established relationship.

Consider the case of Trina. She learns that she is HIV positive and decides to share this information with her best friend, Suzi. Suzi is likely to ask how Trina contracted HIV, and this question triggers discussion of the topics of Larry and of the sexual relationship Trina and Larry were having, a fact unknown to Suzi. What Suzi learns may not fit with her current expectations about the roles she and Trina have had together. However, Trina's disclosure of this news to her good friend reinforces the importance of and the emotional support from the relationship. Fortunately, at sensitive moments like this between two good friends, each draws on her well-developed understanding of the role expectations and behaves in keeping with these expectations. It is rare, for example, for Suzi to announce to Trina, following disclosure of her HIV status and her sexual relationship with Larry, that she is ending the relationship with Trina. More likely, she will show great support and probably great emotion, in part because she too is confused by this sudden news and about how to incorporate it into her expectations about Trina and about their future relationship. From Trina's viewpoint, the support and emotion are much-needed reinforcements that reaffirm the relationship and the roles. Both understand that the future holds unknowns but also that they will work through the new realities together, drawing on the reservoir of support, respect, and love.

While the disclosure situation with good friends generally proceeds in this manner, this is not always the case with more casual friends, work colleagues, and family. Let us consider the case of casual friends and work colleagues first; families require special attention. The role experiences and expectations we develop with casual friends or work colleagues usually are much more limited and less complex than the roles we develop with good, close friends. We may, for example, work very well with a particular colleague, precisely because we have carefully circumscribed our role interrelationships. Indeed, we can have good work relationships with people with whom we disagree on important social or political issues by limiting the dimensions of our roles with them.

It is these very limitations, however, that present the challenge for an HIV-positive individual regarding disclosure of HIV status. The HIV-positive individual is not sure whether the role expectations can incorporate the news of HIV or even whether the role expectations will preclude an immediate, negative reaction, in contrast to the superficially pleasant demeanor that is part of the roles most of us have with casual friends and colleagues. However, there is the great potential for a significant expansion and deepening of the role expectations with particular individuals, such as a work colleague who now discloses that her husband is HIV positive or a casual friend who discloses that he has been HIV positive for several years.

The problem for the HIV-positive individual is that he or she cannot know in advance how the limited role expectations with casual friends or colleagues will accommodate the news of HIV-positive status. In all likelihood, the HIV-positive individual will take cautious steps toward greater disclosure, wanting to avoid rejection or negative reactions that would only add to the pressure on self-esteem as discussed above.

We said that families need special consideration. We are born into family roles of son or daughter, brother or sister, which are laden with expectations and defined through intense experiences as we grow up. The extent of the son/daughter and brother/sister role expectations varies for each of us, and the centrality of these to our own self-concept also varies greatly. These roles are very important to some of us, with interrelationships similar to those we described above for close friends. Others of us are less involved in these particular roles, with interrelationships more like those with work colleagues. Because of these variations, some newly identified HIV-positive individuals will consult their families first, while others will avoid telling their families this news until absolutely necessary—and perhaps not even then.

Accepting the Reality of Infection

Each HIV-positive individual eventually begins to accept the reality of HIV infection. In different ways for each individual, the self-concept is adjusted and roles are changed. The process of acceptance involves a reshaping of the individual's self-concept and self-schema and a reassessment of role expectations and responsibilities.

This process of cognitive and role adjustments involves both risks and opportunities. The risks include dealing with issues such as unresolved tensions in relationships, unrealistic hopes and dreams, unattainable goals, and unpleasant personality dimensions. There are opportunities as well, some very significant. As HIV-positive individuals reshape their self-concept, they are able to focus on their strengths and anchor their goals in ways that are most satisfying to them. No longer, for example, must they strive to achieve goals that became incorporated into their self-concept through pressure from family and others but were not truly their own. HIV-positive individuals also have the opportunity to leave unsatisfying roles and adopt new roles. Some of these new roles might include public presentations to groups about HIV; work with people with AIDS in their terminal phases; volunteer work on causes that are important to them; or more individual but equally satisfying roles such as amateur artist, gardener, or daily exercise walker.

The process of adjustment is usually not easy and, for many HIV-positive individuals, is one that is never completely resolved. The irregular and unpredictable pattern of positive and negative physiological changes that occur over the course of seropositivity can give the HIV-positive individual renewed hope one day and dejection the next. In this respect, those with HIV and AIDS are similar to those with other life-threatening diseases like cancer. Kübler-Ross[2] identified five stages through which many patients with fatal conditions progress: denial, anger, bargaining, depression, and acceptance.

We have already illustrated the first stage, denial, in our discussion of Fernando. This stage is followed by anger at having this life-threatening condition. Sometimes this anger is directed at particular people whom the individual blames for causing them to have this condition or at people with whom the individual has old grudges and complaints unrelated to their illness. Other times, the anger is more diffuse and nonspecific; it can be focused at the world in general or at those who happen to be around the individual. In this latter case, the individual unintentionally hurts those closest to him or her and inadvertently threatens their continued support and understanding. Those around the individual need to be prepared for this behavior and realize that they are being scapegoated and not personally targeted.

The third stage, bargaining, involves moderating the angry feelings and accepting parts of the diagnosis, while at the same time hoping that other parts can be "traded away" in exchange for "good" behavior, hard work, serious effort, good intentions, or the like. When the futility of bargaining becomes clear, depression sets in. The individual realizes that the new reality is uncompromising and unchangeable. Finally, in the fifth stage—acceptance—the full reality of the disease settles in and the individual accepts this reality in both its good and bad aspects.

We should point out that not everyone progresses through all of these stages and that there is no inevitability to the stages. Rather, the stages were a useful characterization of the progression of acceptance of disease by many individuals with a variety of life-threatening diseases. These stages are generally applicable to the case of HIV and AIDS, although, due to the stigma associated with AIDS, there have been some variations in the way the stages are experienced and dealt with by some of those who are HIV positive or who have AIDS. To understand this difference, consider those diagnosed with breast cancer, for example. These people are not stigmatized (that is, judged negatively) solely on the basis of having cancer. They do not lose their jobs or their lodging because they have a cancer diagnosis. Those who are HIV positive or diagnosed with AIDS are, too often, treated differently: They are judged and even censured by some people for having the disease, they might be fired from their job, or they might lose their lodging. There have been and, unfortunately, continue to be, instances where those with HIV have their houses set on fire or are physically attacked because of their HIV status.

The constant possibility of rejection, by those in general society, of individuals who are HIV positive or have AIDS affects the progress of these individuals through the stages of acceptance. This can be illustrated by two examples, one with an individual focus and one with a group focus.

Greg Louganis: An Individual Dilemma

U.S. Olympian Greg Louganis was the winner of double gold medals in diving at both the 1984 and 1988 Olympic Games. In 1988, at the start of the Olympic trials, Louganis knew that he was HIV positive.[3] Louganis had accepted this reality and moved beyond it. He focused all his energy and attention on the 1988 competition, knowing that he was not at his peak physiological performance level (due to aging, not to HIV status). Louganis was comfortable enough with his HIV status to share this with his coach but not with others, due in large part to the strong stigma associated with HIV and AIDS in the late 1980s. In addition, he believed his HIV status was irrelevant to the conditions of a diving competition (the Olympic Committee required no disclosure of HIV status for any athletes at that time and still does not), and he believed that he would not put anyone else involved in the diving competition at risk.

During the diving competition, Louganis hit his head on the diving board, cut his scalp, and bled into the pool as he tumbled into the water. Louganis had never considered this possibility but immediately realized the risk his bleeding cut could present to the team doctor who was about to put temporary stitches in his scalp so that he could continue the competition. He also wondered about the risk to other divers from the blood in the pool. (Louganis need not have worried about the latter issue; the chlorine in a swimming pool quickly kills HIV, which would have been greatly diluted in any case by the water.)

From our earlier discussions of self-concept and self-esteem, we can see how Louganis was faced with strong and complex psychological pressures in deciding whether to tell the doctor his HIV status. On the one hand, he could reveal his HIV status and refuse to let the doctor sew his scalp. This would throw the diving competition into turmoil (and, to some extent, the entire Olympic Games) and end the possibility that he would win a record-breaking second set of gold medals (he had 20 minutes to be back on the board for his next dive). Like other Olympic competitors, Louganis's self-concept and self-esteem were overwhelmingly tied to his competitive ability and success. Forfeiting his opportunity to set another Olympic record would be a great blow to his self-concept. In addition, disclosing his HIV status in such a public manner to people around the world and the censure he probably would have to endure would further undermine his self-esteem. On the other hand, Louganis could say nothing and not reveal his HIV status to the doctor. This would put the doctor at potential risk for HIV. With all of these conflicting and complex psychological pressures and in a dazed physiological state from the blow to his head, Louganis later said he was "paralyzed with fear" and so he said nothing.

The team doctor was going through his own risk assessment and decision making (see Chapter 8). He thought about using plastic gloves for protection, but he knew there were none available and that he had only 10 minutes to complete the stitching by the time he completed his exam. He made the decision to proceed with caution. (The doctor correctly knew that touching HIV-infected blood alone is not a sufficient condition for HIV transmission; he would have had to have opened up a path of transmission by cutting or pricking himself. See Chapter 7.) The doctor subsequently tested HIV negative.

Louganis went on to win double gold medals, but he also had to deal with new uneasiness about the realities of HIV infection. Since 1988, Louganis has kept this uneasiness to himself and a very small group of friends. By releasing his autobiography, in which he acknowledges publicly that he is not only HIV positive but also has AIDS, Louganis moved to another, deeper level of acceptance of the reality of infection. By publicly sharing this information, Louganis hoped to send a message to others about the need to stop HIV infection and the personal agonies due to the stigma still associated with HIV and AIDS.

ACT UP: A Collective Response

The acceptance of the reality of infection takes many forms for those with HIV. While the five stages described above are generally applicable, the anger stage in particular can be experienced very differently by someone with AIDS as contrasted with someone with another life-threatening disease but without the social stigma (such as cancer).

The explicit and implicit rejection that the HIV-positive person experiences can provide additional fuel for the person's anger, beyond the normal anger that arises inside the person in confronting any life-threatening condition. Because the rejection arises from the misguided fear and unfounded prejudice of others (subjects to which we will soon turn), the HIV-positive individual is understandably frustrated by and angry at actions that are unfair and unjust. For some HIV-positive people, their personal anger at having a life-threatening disease is infused and overtaken by the "rational" anger arising from insensitive statements and discriminatory actions. The resulting feelings of anger and injustice in some HIV-positive individuals have provided powerful fuel for actions of different types and, in some cases, with unusual effectiveness. These transformations of anger into action provide one example of the kinds of unique opportunities PWAs have to effect change.

Consider, for instance, the emergence of the ACT UP organizations in the United States and later abroad. ACT UP originally stood for "AIDS Coalition to Unleash Power." Now, it is more generally associated with groups of PWAs or their supporters who organize and implement public demonstrations to increase awareness of AIDS issues. Their tactics are usually tough: chaining themselves to government buildings, disrupting a church service, throwing vials of blood-like substances, and chalking outlines of dead people on public sidewalks. These actions usually involve a public display of anger and a confounding, if not an outright rejection, of role expectations. As we have discussed, sudden, one-sided changes in role activities and expectations are quite uncomfortable for those involved in social interaction. These changes, however, get people's attention, and ACT UP has not missed this opportunity to raise people's consciousness about AIDS by jarring and challenging role expectations and experiences.

Consider one famous ACT UP church demonstration, which occurred in New York City at the Catholic cathedral. Demonstrations during church services (including such activities as shouting, passing out information, and lying on the floor) are not part of most people's role expectations of how those attending Catholic church services should behave. Imagine the attention the small group of ACT UP demonstrators received—as well as the anger they generated—when they began their demonstration. The media covered the event, which was broadcast around the world; there even was a documentary film made about the planning for and the execution of the demonstration.

At the individual ACT UP demonstrator level, this event provided a vehicle for release of personal anger and for action in the service of greater AIDS awareness. For the individual, non-ACT UP church-goer, the event provoked reactions from irritation to frustration and anger. At the larger community level, the demonstrators accomplished at least one of their goals—greater attention to AIDS in New York, in the United States, and around the world—but whether they gained more than they lost in public support was unclear. Even among the New York City ACT UP group, the decision to hold the church demonstration was controversial and not endorsed by everyone.

Other ACT UP–motivated activities have had more clearly positive community outcomes. Members of ACT UP and other AIDS activist organizations pressured the National Institutes of Health (NIH) in Washington, D.C., to speed up the official approval process for potentially lifesaving drugs and therapies. As they pointed out, in polite meetings with NIH officials and in not-so-polite demonstrations in front of NIH headquarters, they were dying and they could not wait for the 5- to 10-year-long process. The AIDS activists wanted to be allowed to make the decision themselves whether to participate in experimental therapies. NIH expanded its procedures for approval of new drugs and, in some instances, now allows greater availability of potentially beneficial drugs through local physicians in community-based trials.

These examples demonstrate some of the larger-scale opportunities open to HIV-positive individuals as they progress in dealing with the realities of HIV infection. There are many smaller-scale opportunities as well, which include such activities as speaking on panels about HIV and AIDS or working in volunteer jobs with community groups on activities related to HIV and

AIDS or on unrelated activities, such as education or environmental protection. In addition to the benefits to others from these large- and small-scale actions, there are benefits to the HIV-positive individual in increased self-esteem from achievements in new roles.

SOCIETAL DIMENSIONS OF HIV AND AIDS

We have been focusing on PWAs—people living directly with AIDS and HIV. Now, we want to expand the focus beyond PWAs, to everyone else who is living with HIV and AIDS. We will concentrate here on two general issues—prejudice and discrimination—which underlie many of society's specific actions related to HIV and AIDS, such as insurance regulations, health-care policies, and laws related to HIV and AIDS. We will illustrate the general principles with two examples of these specific actions: laws related to injection drug users and health-care practices.

Prejudice

Prejudice is an unfavorable attitude toward a group of people. It arises from schemas that people have created that are associated with particular groups of individuals. Racial or ethnic groups are common targets for prejudices because their members have easily identifiable common characteristics and because there has been a history of friction between different groups.

Negative stereotypes form the cognitive basis for prejudices. Stereotypes are group-based schemas, as contrasted with individual-based schemas (such as, for example, your schema about your mother). Stereotypes can be either positive or negative, but, like our other social schemas, they usually reflect society's general appraisal of the object of the stereotypes. For example, our stereotype of newborn babies is quite positive: cute, content, cuddly objects. (If you doubt the power of this stereotype, try telling a new mother that her baby is not cute, is ill-tempered, and repels you.) At the other extreme, our stereotype of vagrants is negative: shiftless, ill-kept, bad-tempered, dangerous people. (If you want to test the power of this stereotype, try reacting in a very obviously positive manner to vagrants on the street in the presence of "regular" community members; you likely will be the butt of negative comments from these passers-by.)

Because they are group based, stereotypes are usually not accurate in their details when applied to individual members of the group. Not all newborn babies are cute and not all vagrants are bad tempered. When we have opportunities to interact with particular individuals (our brother's new baby, for example, or the vagrant we always run into in the park), we can develop individually based schemas that may begin with the stereotype but are changed to relate to the specific individual. The original stereotypes are usually not changed to accommodate the new, individual-specific experience unless we have many experiences with many new babies or many vagrants. You may have heard people say something like, "Sam is a nice guy down on his luck; he's the exception that proves the [vagrant] rule." This explanation resolves the apparent contradiction between the positive appraisal of Sam and the negative appraisal associated with the vagrant stereotype; it also reinforces the negative evaluation of vagrants.

With this general background, let us consider the relationship of prejudice to HIV and AIDS. To do so, think back to 1981. Although not yet labeled, HIV and AIDS first appeared in reports about unusual life-threatening diseases in homosexual men (see Chapter 1). As the epidemic grew in the next few years, more and more male homosexuals died and the general population came to learn of HIV and AIDS.

How did the community react to the news of these strange deaths? As we learned in the first part of this chapter, when new information arises, people draw on relevant cognitive schemas to interpret the information. Schemas related to death and dying prematurely were probably activated for most people, causing some fear in most people. In addition, other related schemas were probably activated, such as those related to homosexual men. For most people, these latter schemas are based on no direct contact with homosexual men but instead on stereotypes, which are generally negative in our society at the present and were even more negative at the outset of the AIDS epidemic.

Prejudice against homosexuals initially fueled the reaction of the general populace to HIV and AIDS. For these people, a negative outcome (death) was occurring to a negatively evaluated group (homosexuals); consequently, it was easy to blame the victims of HIV and AIDS for their deaths. As the epidemic spread into the injection drug-using community, prejudice against this particular community by the general population further fueled the negative reaction to HIV and AIDS. By blaming these victims, people in the general population could explain HIV and AIDS as originating from these "bad" people. This relieved them of any fear that they would get AIDS (since they were not members of these negatively stereotyped groups) and also relieved them of any responsibility for action toward these victims (since the victims had brought this on themselves).

As AIDS began to affect positively stereotyped groups, the situation became more cognitively confusing, and it was more difficult for people to reconcile the positive and negative aspects of their schemas. Babies were born with AIDS and hemophiliac children developed AIDS. Because of the positive stereotypes associated with these groups, these PWAs were not blamed but instead were called "innocent victims"; it was not their fault that they had AIDS. Then, favorite movie and TV stars began to die from AIDS and esteemed sports figures announced that they were HIV positive. For some people, the AIDS epidemic was brought even closer: a colleague at work reported that he was HIV positive or the daughter of their next-door neighbor became sick with AIDS opportunistic infections.

As HIV and AIDS have spread throughout society, it has become more difficult for most people to use negative stereotypes of certain groups to explain the epidemic, to distance themselves from it, and to justify inaction. However, there is still a general prejudice in the population against those with HIV and AIDS. This prejudice exerts a strong influence on societal actions and policies related to HIV and AIDS and frequently results in discrimination.

Discrimination

Prejudice relates to attitudes; discrimination relates to actions. Discrimination is any behavior toward an individual based only on the individual's membership in a particular group. In social terms, discrimination is usually thought of as only negative actions and we will use it with this connotation. However, be aware that positive discrimination is also possible: favoritism shown to an individual based solely on group membership.

The operation of HIV and AIDS discrimination can be best seen in specific examples, since discrimination involves concrete actions and behaviors related to specific contexts and issues. We will consider two examples: laws related to HIV prevention programs for injection drug users and health-care practices for those with HIV and AIDS.

HIV Prevention Programs for Injection Drug Users

As discussed in Chapters 7 and 9, we know how to prevent the transmission of HIV infection among injection drug users: Remove the possibility of transporting HIV-infected blood from one person to another. Drug users can accomplish this either by not sharing needles or by cleaning their needles before reuse. The challenge for many drug users is that they cannot buy clean needles, do not have the resources to buy them (even if available), or do not have the materials or time to clean needles before reuse. Those working in HIV prevention with drug users have recommended "harm reduction" strategies and, in particular, have advocated clean needle-exchange programs. In these programs, drug users can exchange used needles for new ones at no cost and with no questions asked. A large-scale evaluation of a set of needle-exchange programs was recently completed by the American Foundation for AIDS Research; it provided conclusive proof of the effectiveness of needle-exchange programs in significantly reducing rates of new HIV infection.

Unfortunately, discrimination is preventing the implementation of these successful programs. Only a few cities, with special exemptions granted by local officials, have instituted these needle-exchange programs. Repeatedly, legislators vote down or elected officials veto new laws which would permit these programs. The legislators and officials say that their constituents do not want laws that endorse drug use. In fact, the proposed laws carefully avoid any such endorsement and focus only on the exchange as a means of stopping the transmission of HIV. Some proposed laws have even included provisions to increase resources for drug treatment and cessation programs. The underlying problem is general prejudice against drug users, which results in discriminatory actions. Most people in society do not support using drugs and, therefore, do not support any actions that would benefit drug users. Some people are so prejudiced that they are comfortable with the status quo: letting drug users share infected needles and increase their risk of HIV.

How can this situation be changed? As we know from our discussion in Chapter 9, changing a person's attitudes and behaviors related to his or her own personal HIV risk is difficult; changing a person's attitudes and behaviors related to others' HIV risk is as difficult. In the case of drug users, we would need to educate the general public in much more detail about the reasons for and realities of drug use. It is unlikely that someone who is unsympathetic to drug users would pay much attention to our educational program. Alternatively, we could try to explain how ignoring the drug-using community only causes other problems (such as increased crime and violence) and results in costly actions (such as more police). Again, it will be difficult to convey this message to someone who has already made up his or her mind and has a strong stereotype to justify it. The most productive approach will probably be the slow expansion of the successful pilot programs developed in several cities. As the benefits become clearer, more people may be willing to support a harm-reduction strategy, which at least improves one part of the drug-use picture.

Health-Care Practices

Unlike the previous example, the story of discrimination in health-care practices has a more positive outcome. At the outset of the AIDS epidemic, however, there were numerous examples of discrimination against those with HIV and AIDS by health- care workers and institutions. Some workers refused to treat those with AIDS; others did so but with insensitivity and, in some instances, outright hostility. Health-care workers are not required to treat everyone who comes to them; generally, the law is that treatment cannot be refused in "emergencies." Because of the flexibility in interpretation of who and what should be treated and what is an "emergency," discrimination against those with HIV and AIDS can play a role in decisions by health-care workers, sometimes blatantly and other times more subtly.

Currently, the situation is greatly improved from that at the outset of the AIDS epidemic, although it is not completely without problems. Part of the reason for this is the increase in our knowledge base of HIV and AIDS. Unlike the situation at the outset of the epidemic in the early 1980s, we know how HIV is transmitted and how transmission can be prevented. Also, universal precautions are now in general practice for health-care workers who can be exposed to potentially infected body fluids, whether the agent is HIV, hepatitis, or other infectious agents. These changes have lessened the fear of HIV infection among health-care workers and reduced the psychological pressure to take actions that protect the health-care worker at the expense of the patient.

The AIDS epidemic has even fostered the development of new health-care approaches, such as hospice care for those in the terminal stages of AIDS. Typically, those in the terminal stages of an illness are in a hospital intensive care unit, receiving a variety of medical services, many very costly and of dubious value in prolonging the patient's life. Daily costs in an intensive care unit can be in excess of $1,500 a day. Hospice is an alternative for those in the final stages of a terminal illness. Hospice care, first developed in England, primarily involves the management of pain so the patient can live comfortably in the final stage of life. Hospice care (where daily costs are in the $150 to $250 range) is typically given in the patient's home or a home-like facility and involves a team of care-givers, including those with medical, social, and, if appropriate, spiritual expertise. The focus of attention is not just the patient but includes his or her closest family and friends, who themselves become active care-givers. While hospice existed prior to AIDS, the AIDS crisis provided a catalyst for its development as a more humane and cost-effective approach to care during the terminal stage.

In this chapter, we have presented two frameworks to assist in understanding the human and societal dimensions of the AIDS epidemic: the cognitive perspective and the role perspective. The most important and relevant dimensions are and will continue to be different for each of us, including those directly affected by HIV and those more distantly affected but involved in societal decisions about actions toward those with HIV and AIDS. As new human and societal dimensions of AIDS develop, the cognitive and role perspectives can be useful anchors not only to understand these aspects but also to deal with them and, in the best cases, capitalize on opportunities for positive change.

Notes

1. The discussion here is based on K. Deaux, F. C. Dane, and L. S. Wrightsman, *Social Psychology in the '90s*. 6th Edition. Pacific Grove, Calif.: Brooks/Cole, 1993. The reader is encouraged to consult this book for fuller discussions of social psychological theories and concepts presented in this chapter.

2. E. Kübler-Ross. *On Death and Dying*. New York: Macmillan, 1969. Also see E. Kübler-Ross. *AIDS: The Ultimate Challenge*. New York: Macmillan, 1987.

3. See Greg Louganis's autobiography for more details: *Breaking the Surface*. New York: Random House, 1995.

Chapter 11

Future Directions in Combating AIDS

FUTURE DIRECTIONS FOR BIOMEDICAL EFFORTS

- Prevention of Infection
- Treatment of Infected Individuals

FUTURE DIRECTIONS FOR SOCIAL EFFORTS

- Education
- Research

A FINAL NOTE OF OPTIMISM: TIME IS ON OUR SIDE

In this book, we have learned about AIDS in terms of both basic biomedical and social aspects. In terms of the biomedical picture, we have considered the virus (HIV), the immune system, the physical manifestations of AIDS, and transmission of the virus. From the social perspective, we have explored individual risk assessment, the prevention of HIV transmission, and the human and societal aspects of AIDS. However, the fact remains that HIV infection is continuing to spread in many areas of the world, and there is currently no cure for the disease. How can we respond to this disease, and what are the areas where we are likely to see activity and progress?

FUTURE DIRECTIONS FOR BIOMEDICAL EFFORTS

The biomedical community will focus on two major problems regarding AIDS: (1)*prevention of infection through vaccines* and (2) *treatment of infected individuals who develop symptoms of the disease.* Let's look at some of the areas where current and future efforts are likely to focus.

Prevention of Infection

Research

Remarkable progress has been made in terms of biomedical research on AIDS in finding and studying the virus itself. Currently, the lack of a convenient animal model system is a major stumbling block. Faster progress could be made in understanding the disease process and testing therapies if HIV caused a similar disease in experimental animals. However, HIV only infects man and higher apes, such as chimpanzees; furthermore, the virus does not cause disease in chimpanzees. Several retroviruses similar to HIV have been found recently in monkeys (SIV), and one strain induces immunodeficiency in rhesus monkeys, so this may be a useful model system. However, monkeys are very expensive to maintain in laboratories, they are in short supply, and the use of primates in research is strongly opposed by some animal welfare advocates. Thus, other more convenient animal model systems are desirable. One possibility is cats: There are two retroviruses of cats that cause immunodeficiencies. One of these cat viruses (FIV) is a lentivirus.

Recently, it has been possible to grow cells of the human immune system in special mice. These mice carry a genetic defect called *severe combined immunodeficiency (SCID)*, which leaves them with crippled immune systems—much like those in AIDS patients. Because SCID mice lack functional cellular immunity, it is possible to implant them with human cells without tissue rejection taking place. Researchers have recently developed techniques to implant human fetal tissues containing stem cells for the blood into SCID mice. It is then possible to reconstitute these mice with functional human immune cells, including T-lymphocytes and B-lymphocytes. They have also found that if these SCID mice are infected by HIV, the virus will establish infection in the human tissue and destroy the T_{helper} lymphocytes, just as it does in humans. Thus, it may be possible to study some of the mechanisms by which HIV attacks the immune system in these mice. In addition, they may be very useful for testing potential antiviral drugs.

Vaccines

Ideally, the most effective prevention of HIV infection would be a vaccine that blocks virus infection in an individual. Indeed, effective vaccines have been developed against most human viruses that cause serious diseases. While several different possible vaccines against HIV are under development, there are some theoretical reasons why it may be difficult to develop an effective one. As discussed in Chapter 4, HIV has a unique ability to evade the immune system in an infected individual. Briefly, this results from (1) the high mutation rate of the virus, particularly in the *env* gene; (2) the ability of the virus to establish a latent state in some cells; and (3) the ability of the virus to spread by cell-to-cell contact. The object of a vaccine is to raise a protective immune response to the infectious agent. Since HIV evades the immune system so efficiently, it may be difficult for a vaccine to prevent HIV infection in an individual even if it can induce production of neutralizing antibodies or cell-mediated immunity.

Despite these theoretical concerns, a number of HIV vaccines are under development. Most of these vaccines have been developed by state-of-the-art gene splicing (or recombinant DNA) techniques that have allowed large-scale production of individual viral proteins. The predominant HIV proteins that make up these potential vaccines are *env* proteins (for instance, gp120) and, to a lesser extent, *gag* proteins. In addition, inactivated whole HIV virus is being tested. Most of these vaccines can raise anti-HIV antibody responses when injected into monkeys or humans. Planning for a U.S. government-sponsored vaccine trial in humans is taking place, and several different vaccines will probably be compared, if the societal concerns (such as those discussed in Chapter 10) can be resolved.

Considerable HIV vaccine research has focused on simian immunodeficiency viruses (SIVs) since they are closely related to HIV, and some SIV strains cause AIDS in certain monkey species. As mentioned above, chimpanzees are the only monkeys that HIV can infect, but the virus does not cause AIDS in these animals. Thus, many principles of HIV vaccines are being studied by developing analogous vaccines for SIV and testing their abilities to inhibit both SIV infection and disease in monkeys. Using the SIV model system, vaccines against individual SIV proteins have not been very effective. A vaccine consisting of killed SIV virus particles has also been prepared. When this killed virus was used to immunize monkeys, it prevented them from developing viral infection or immunodeficiency when injected with low doses of live SIV virus. While this was encouraging, this vaccine only worked with low virus doses. Moreover, it could not protect from infection if live SIV-infected cells were injected—a situation probably closer to natural routes of HIV infection.

Very recent experiments with the SIV model system raise the prospects for an attenuated live virus vaccine—analogous to the live poliovirus vaccine (Sabin vaccine) commonly used today. Researchers inactivated one of the SIV accessory genes (*nef*; see Chapter 4), and they showed that this mutant SIV could still infect monkeys, but it does not induce disease. Moreover, prior infection with the *nef*-mutant SIV could efficiently protect monkeys from infection by normal SIV, and these monkeys did not develop immunodeficiency. The immunity induced by *nef*-mutant SIV was much stronger than that induced by the killed virus vaccine. HIV has a *nef* gene as well, which raises the possibility of generating a live, attenuated *nef*-mutant HIV as a vaccine. In this case, safety considerations will be very important.

As we discussed in Chapter 3, there are two branches of the immune system: the humoral immune system produces antibody molecules, while the cellular immune system produces antigen-specific T-lymphocytes. Due to intricacies of the immune system, most of the anti-HIV vaccines currently being tested are likely to induce anti-HIV antibody responses. However, if cellular immunity to HIV is important for resistance to HIV infection, these vaccines may not be effective. A few vaccines designed to induce cellular immunity to HIV are under development as well. The first of these is about to undergo human trials.

In all cases, the first steps for vaccine trials will simply determine if individuals injected with the test vaccines produce antibodies (or other immune responses) against HIV and if they experience no other harmful side effects. In the initial trials, the proper doses of vaccine to give an immune response are also determined. Once this has been established, then other, large-scale trials will test if the vaccines are effective in preventing HIV infection. Some of the vaccines are currently moving through the vital clinical trial phases.

Testing an HIV vaccine in humans brings together scientific and societal issues, as discussed in Chapter 10. Because of the bioethical issues involved in using humans, groups of specialists in both the biomedical and psychological aspects of HIV and AIDS are working together to implement trials that take scientific, human, and societal considerations into account.

Treatment of Infected Individuals

Biomedical efforts to treat HIV-infected individuals will focus on three main areas: (1) *antivirals* that interfere with continued HIV infection, (2) *restoration of the immune system,* and (3) *treatments of opportunistic infections and cancers.*

Antivirals

As described in Chapters 4 and 6, AZT, which is an antiviral compound against HIV, is an effective drug in AIDS patients. The fact that this drug works means that agents that interfere with continued HIV infection in an AIDS patient will improve the clinical status. Thus, great efforts are being made to develop other antiviral compounds that will also block HIV infection. Ultimately, it may be possible to use several antivirals in combination and completely block the spread of HIV infection in an individual.

As was discussed in Chapter 4, AZT works by specifically blocking DNA synthesis carried out by HIV reverse transcriptase. Other related compounds are also being tested to see if they specifically affect HIV reverse transcriptase. Such compounds might have equivalent antiviral effects. If they have fewer side effects than AZT, they may be even more effective in treating HIV-infected individuals. As described in Chapter 5, two additional antivirals related to AZT have recently been approved for anti-HIV therapy: dideoxyinosine (DDI) and dideoxycytosine (DDC). These drugs are predominantly recommended for individuals who cannot tolerate AZT or for whom

AZT has ceased to be effective. While they are effective against HIV, they also have side effects. Nevertheless, they may be important because AZT does not indefinitely reduce the amount of virus in HIV-infected individuals.

In addition to drugs such as AZT, other antivirals targeted at reverse transcriptase are also being developed. As described in Chapter 4, AZT (and its relatives DDI and DDC) inhibits HIV replication by mimicking normal building blocks of DNA and being selectively incorporated by reverse transcriptase into viral DNA as opposed to cellular DNA. Viral DNA that has incorporated these compounds cannot be completed, and virus replication is aborted. Other compounds have been developed that directly inhibit the activity of HIV reverse transcriptase, with relatively little effect on cellular DNA polymerases. The net effect of these compounds also is to selectively inhibit HIV replication. One class of reverse transcriptase inhibitors currently being tested is referred to as TIBO inhibitors. TIBO is an abbreviation for the chemical structure of the inhibitory compound.

Another approach to increasing the effectiveness of antiviral therapy is to use combinations of compounds. This principle has been widely exploited in chemotherapy for cancer.

Other potential antivirals are under development, which attack other viral Achilles heels—processes that are vital to the virus but that are not necessary for the survival of the host cell. There are actually nine or ten different genes carried by HIV that specify proteins necessary for the virus's life cycle. Any of these viral proteins are potential targets for new antiviral drugs. One viral protein that is being intensively investigated as a target for antiviral therapy is *protease*, another product of the *pol* gene (see Chapter 4). Recent advances in research on HIV protease have included purification of large amounts of the protein and determination of its three-dimensional structure. This has allowed pharmaceutical researchers to design a series of compounds that specifically inhibit HIV protease (and viral replication) with little effect on similar enzymes in normal cells. Several protease inhibitors are being tested in clinical trials on HIV-infected people. Other viral proteins that are being investigated as targets for antiviral therapy include the *tat* and *rev* regulatory proteins. Currently, at least two compounds that inhibit HIV *tat* activity have been developed, and they are undergoing clinical trials. A potential advantage of antivirals targeted at *tat* and *rev* is that these compounds might prevent expression of HIV in cells even if they have already been infected and contain integrated viral DNA. Basic research on the growth cycle of HIV and related viruses will be important in pointing out new antivirals.

Another potential class of antivirals is those that interfere with the ability of the virus to enter cells. If the virus entry process is inhibited, then spread of infection within an individual might be inhibited. As discussed in Chapter 4, HIV virus particles initially attach to cells by way of the cellular receptor for CD4 protein, which is imbedded in the surface of normal T-lymphocytes and macrophages. Recently, recombinant DNA techniques have been used to make large amounts of a part of pure CD4 protein. Test-tube experiments have shown that if this CD4 protein fragment is incubated with T-lymphocytes or macrophages, it can saturate all the CD4 receptors and prevent subsequent infection with HIV. It is possible that this approach might be effective in people as well.

Another compound that sparked great interest a year or two ago is called *dextran sulfate*. Test-tube experiments showed that dextran sulfate can also block HIV infection by interfering with viral entry, although the mechanism of action is not understood. Dextran sulfate is currently licensed for use as a blood anticoagulant in other countries, such as Japan, which means that the drug has been successfully tested in those countries for lack of side effects. However, clinical trials did not show dramatic results in the ability of dextran sulfate to reduce HIV in infected individuals. Thus, interest in it has waned.

As time passes, new potential antivirals continually appear—some from pharmaceutical laboratories and some from nontraditional sources. They initially spark great interest, typically based on anecdotal reports of effectiveness. It is important to subject these compounds to rigorous scientific testing (clinical trials; see Chapter 6 for AZT) to determine if they work as claimed. If not, they could worsen the conditions of HIV and AIDS patients who abandon traditional and proven therapies in favor of the new compounds. Recently, one compound that attracted considerable interest was GLQ223, or Compound Q. This drug is derived from a Chinese herbal medicine (from bitter cucumber) and it was found to kill HIV-infected cells in culture. However, standard clinical trials have not definitively proven GLQ223's effectiveness. In addition, serious neurological side effects, including coma, have occurred in some individuals taking GLQ223 in early clinical trials. Thus, interest in this compound has declined for the time being.

Two new classes of potential antiviral agents have recently been developed out of basic molecular biology research. One class of compounds is called *antisense* molecules. These are small pieces of single-stranded DNA or RNA that can specifically form double-stranded complexes with HIV viral RNA, similar in structure to double-stranded DNA. Formation of these double-stranded complexes can lead to destruction of the viral RNA. As a result, an infected cell cannot produce viral RNA, viral protein, or virus particles. Current research is focused on establishing methods to effectively deliver these antisense molecules to infected cells and determining which antisense molecules (directed against which regions of the viral RNA) are most effective. The other class of potential antiviral compounds is called ribozymes. Ribozymes are very specialized antisense RNA molecules. When they combine with HIV RNA, they attack the HIV RNA and cause cutting at particular sites. Thus, they can inactivate virus expression.

Restoration of the Immune System

Most of the clinical symptoms in AIDS result from failure of the immune system, due to depletion of T_{helper} lymphocytes. If the immunological defects can be repaired, then the disease might be arrested or even reversed. As discussed in Chapter 3, all cells of the blood (including those of the immune system) arise by division and differentiation from stem cells that are located in the bone marrow. This process is controlled by a complex series of growth factors which circulate in the body, as described in Chapter 3. Blood cell growth factors are currently the subjects of a great deal of research—they are important in many other diseases in addition to AIDS. Ultimately, it may be possible to use these growth factors to stimulate and regenerate the immune system in AIDS patients. Of course, it will be important to use these growth factors in conjunction with antivirals. Otherwise, continued HIV infection would destroy the immune system again. Another potential complication is that growth factors may directly or indirectly activate HIV from latently infected cells.

In addition to naturally occurring growth factors for the immune system, several artificial substances that may be able to stimulate immune system regeneration are also being developed and tested.

Another possible approach to restoring the immune system would be to supply an AIDS patient with functional T-lymphocytes. Technically, this is very difficult to accomplish because mature T-lymphocytes do not divide. Instead, as described in Chapter 3, it would be necessary to provide new blood stem cells that can divide and differentiate into functional T-lymphocytes. The most logical way to supply these stem cells is to carry out a bone marrow transplant, in which uninfected bone marrow cells are implanted into the recipient individual. These bone marrow cells could then produce functional T-lymphocytes. The greatest technical problem with this approach is that HIV in the infected individual can infect the transplanted bone marrow and destroy the resulting T-lymphocytes. Current cutting-edge research is focused on developing ways to make bone marrow cells resistant to HIV before transplanting them—for instance, by implanting them with an anti-HIV ribozyme (see above).

Treatment of Opportunistic Infections and Cancers

The major practical problems for AIDS patients generally are the opportunistic infections (OIs) and cancers that result from the lack of immunological protection. Thus, development of better therapies for these OIs and cancers will play an important role in improved treatment of AIDS patients.

In terms of opportunistic infections, it will be necessary to develop effective drugs for each different OI. Many of these infections were rather rare before the AIDS epidemic, since the causative agents generally do not cause disease in healthy individuals. As a result, little effort had been put into developing drugs for them. For example, at present, there is no effective treatment to control cryptosporidiosis as an opportunistic infection. The only recourse right now is to treat the symptoms (diarrhea). Now, much more effort needs to be focused on developing drugs for these OIs.

In addition to developing new drugs, improved methods of delivery are also being developed. As an example, pentamidine is one of two treatments used for pneumocystis pneumonia. Intravenous treatment with pentamidine is the standard procedure, but many patients experience side effects from the drug. Recently, researchers have found that inhalation of a pentamidine mist brings the drug directly to the lungs and is very effective in treating PCP. At the same time, the side effects of the drug are reduced because it is delivered only to the area of infection (the lungs) and not to other regions of the body that may experience side effects. Aerosol pentamidine is now also being used preventively in HIV-infected individuals who have low T_{helper} lymphocyte counts, but who have not yet developed PCP.

The cancers that result from HIV infection range from Kaposi's sarcoma to the tumors of the immune system, called *lymphomas*. These cancers are actually quite distinct diseases and different therapies will be necessary for each of them. In the case of Kaposi's sarcoma, one experimental treatment involves use of a naturally occurring protein called alpha-interferon. Cancer researchers may also provide new therapies for the cancers associated with AIDS.

Treating HIV-infected individuals often involves new or experimental drug therapies. The AIDS crisis has led to some modifications in the typical clinical trial procedures used for licensing drugs in the United States. The FDA oversees drug licensing, and it requires extensive testing in laboratory animals and humans before a drug is approved for therapy. This is a very time-consuming and expensive process, typically taking many years. Largely due to pressure from AIDS activist groups (see Chapter 10), several modifications in these procedures have been developed to speed drug testing and also to make experimental drugs available to patients during the approval process. Traditionally, experimental drugs are only administered through official clinical trials, which usually take place in university research hospitals. To expand the availability of these trials to more patients, *community-based trials* have been established in which experimental drugs are administered to AIDS patients by their local physicians. These physicians then report the results of the treatment to a central source, where the results are pooled.

Another problem with standard clinical trials is that some individuals are too far away from a research university to participate in a trial. As a result, *parallel track* procedures have been developed, in which an experimental drug is made available to a patient (through his or her doctor) in parallel to a clinical trial if that patient is unable to obtain access to the drug otherwise.

Another way AIDS clinical trials have been modified is the development of *surrogate endpoints*. In clinical trials, the standard yardsticks (endpoints) used to judge a drug's effectiveness are development of clinical disease or death. However, this presents a problem for HIV and AIDS, since the time course of infection and disease is so long. When disease or death are used as the endpoints, a clinical trial of an AIDS drug could take many years. As a result, other measurements of an individual's immune system or health have been substituted in preliminary evaluations of HIV drugs. The most common surrogate endpoints are a patient's CD4 (T_{helper}) lymphocyte count and the amount of viral protein (p24 antigen) detectable in the blood. If a drug lowers the amount of circulating viral protein or if it increases the T_{helper} lymphocyte count, it would be provisionally considered effective. In fact, the decisions to approve DDI and DDC as anti-HIV drugs were partly based on clinical trials with surrogate endpoints. However, the accuracy of different surrogate endpoints in reflecting the overall clinical state of HIV-infected individuals is still open to debate.

FUTURE DIRECTIONS FOR SOCIAL EFFORTS

Infectious diseases do not only affect isolated people. On the individual level, the spread of an infectious agent is caused by the interactions of individuals within a society. On the community level, everyone is directly or indirectly living with AIDS. Therefore, in combating infectious diseases, it is important to consider society as a whole in planning solutions. This is particularly important for diseases such as AIDS, for which there is currently no cure or vaccine. Social efforts related to AIDS can make contributions in two main areas: education and research.

Education

There are two aspects of education that can have significant effects on different parts of the AIDS epidemic: education for prevention and education for understanding and compassion.

Education for Prevention

Educational programs targeted to members of high-risk groups will be extremely important. These programs will be the key to making these individuals aware of the dangers they face and also to promoting changes in behavior that will lessen the risks. As described in Chapter 2, the experience with the syphilis epidemic earlier this century shows the effectiveness of proper public health measures. As also discussed in Chapter 2, public health measures effectively limited the last plague outbreak at the turn of this century—even at a time when there was no cure for the disease. This is quite analogous to our present situation with AIDS. As discussed in Chapters 8 and 9, however, changing individual attitudes and behaviors is a challenging task.

In the context of AIDS, public health education has been strongly endorsed by the National AIDS Commission. As discussed in Chapter 7, safer sex recommendations have been developed to reduce the risk of spreading HIV infection through sexual relations. It will be very important to develop effective programs of education and behavior modification to persuade high-risk individuals to adopt safer sex practices. Addressing HIV infection in injection drug users is an extremely critical issue, since these individuals may be the conduit for spread of infection into the general heterosexual population. The current programs have had limited success and they are underfunded.

Development and implementation of public health measures targeted to injection drug users will be challenging. For instance, as mentioned in Chapter 7, there are pilot programs to distribute clean needles to drug addicts, in order to reduce the risk that they will share a contaminated needle with someone else. However, as discussed in Chapter 10, such programs have been opposed by some people who argue that distribution of needles condones and encourages drug addiction.

Development of public health programs to combat AIDS will also require particular attention to ethnic groups. As described in Chapter 6, African Americans and Hispanics represent a disproportionate number of AIDS patients. This is particularly true for HIV-infected individuals who are injection drug users— more than 75 percent of AIDS patients who acquired the disease through injection drug use are African American or Hispanic. Public health programs targeted to these groups will be very important, and they will have to be developed with careful attention to the seven principles described in Chapter 9.

Another important aspect of public health education will be to prevent backsliding in behavior. Behavior modification through public education has clearly been effective in areas where the AIDS epidemic has hit hard—for instance, the gay male community in San Francisco. However, recent follow-up studies have detected a significant frequency of reversion to high-risk sex practices by some men in this community as time has passed. We could have predicted these reversions based on the Precaution-Adoption Process Model discussed in Chapter 9. It will be important to develop methods to promote continued adherence to safer behaviors, even after initial efforts have been effective. We cannot forget the seventh health promotion/disease prevention program principle, the Scientific Principle: All of our programs need to be evaluated on the short- and long-term effects.

Education for Understanding and Compassion

There is another aspect of education that is equally important: educating the general public about HIV, AIDS, and those with the disease. As we discussed in Chapter 10, fear and lack of knowledge and experience have fostered prejudice and discrimination against those with HIV and AIDS. Education of various types and in various forms can help to lessen the fear of HIV and AIDS by increasing knowledge about what HIV is, how it is spread, and how it is medically treated. In addition, as knowledge grows, it will be easier to develop and implement public policies to decrease discrimination against those with HIV and AIDS and to increase programs to stop the spread of the disease.

Health-care workers are another important target for educational efforts. The number of doctors who treat HIV-positive individuals and PWAs has grown, but it still remains small in comparison with the need. Additional educational programs will be necessary to address concerns of doctors and other health-care workers. There are examples of special clinics or wards in hospitals that have made treating PWAs their specialty. In these cases, the quality and sensitivity of care for people living with AIDS has been much better than that generally available. The lessons learned from these settings need to be disseminated to other health-care workers so that more HIV-positive individuals and PWAs can benefit.

From the discussion in Chapter 6, we know that more and more individuals will either be infected with HIV or progress from HIV-positive status to AIDS status. The increases in numbers of individuals affected by the disease will strain our current health-care and social-service systems. In order for the wisest decisions to be made about the allocation of scarce financial and personnel resources, we need to have a general population that is informed about HIV and AIDS. The decisions will be difficult enough without fear and prejudice clouding the public's consideration of options.

Research

All of these education efforts rely on good research. Whether we are developing HIV prevention programs for individuals or AIDS education programs for the general public, we need to draw on the research and theories available to us. For example, as we discussed in Chapter 9, the development of effective HIV prevention programs requires careful and detailed attention to a number of factors (for example, cultural and social aspects of people's situations). Good social research will allow us to identify these factors and determine which approaches will most likely be effective.

We also need to improve our epidemiological and survey research related to AIDS. As AIDS has moved into new communities, our epidemiological research has been slow to catch up. For example, AIDS has begun to appear in the Asian/Pacific Islander community in the United States. Initially, epidemiological data grouped these individuals in the "other" category, instead of the more frequently chosen racial and ethnic categories (Anglo, Hispanic, African American, etc.) Now, Asian/Pacific Islander is listed separately under racial and ethnic groups. As the AIDS epidemic has continued to spread in this community, however, a more detailed breakdown is needed. The cultural practices and beliefs are different enough between Asian/Pacific Islander subgroups that, for effective prevention planning, we need to know more about exactly which subgroups are most affected by HIV.

Likewise, we need accurate survey research on HIV- and AIDS-related knowledge, attitudes, and practices among different segments of the population. We have thorough survey research on certain special study groups of PWAs (for instance, gay men) which has been invaluable in planning and implementing both biomedical and psychosocial programs. Our research on other segments of the population affected by HIV is less complete or missing. For example, we have limited research on injection drug users and their HIV attitudes and practices, and we have very little or almost no systematic research on certain subgroups (such as sex workers) and HIV. Without good research, we are unable to develop a thorough understanding of the HIV-related context and the individuals and factors within it.

Finally, we need better evaluation of all of our HIV and AIDS programs. Only through scientific research can we be sure that we are implementing programs with beneficial effects. Too often, we establish a program with the best of intentions but without a sound scientific plan to assess the actual effects or to detect unintended consequences, both positive and negative. Scientific evaluation provides those working to address the social aspects of AIDS with a way to know if their efforts are effective. Decreases in HIV infection rates are the ultimate outcome of many prevention programs. Unfortunately, we cannot always measure this outcome and, even if we could, HIV infection rates change slowly over a long period of time. For the most complete picture, we need to assess changes in knowledge, attitudes, intentions, practices, and HIV status.

A FINAL NOTE OF OPTIMISM: TIME IS ON OUR SIDE

Many of the facts and statistics about AIDS in this book are quite frightening and depressing, especially since a cure has not been developed yet. Indeed, those who are suffering from the disease or at risk to develop it often express frustration at the apparent lack of progress in AIDS research. But let's look at some time scales to get a sense of perspective. First, as discussed in Chapters 4 and 6, the current estimates are that most HIV-infected individuals will develop AIDS with an average time between initial infection and disease symptoms of eight to ten years. Thus, new therapies and treatments that are developed in the next five or ten years may be able to help many of those who are currently infected.

Second, let's look at the rate of scientific progress in the AIDS epidemic. For comparison, let's consider two other diseases that have had great impacts on society: the ancient disease, plague (Black Death), and the more recent disease, polio (see

Table 11–1
A TIME COMPARISON OF THREE EPIDEMICS

Disease	First Documented Epidemic	Isolation of Agent	First Therapy
Plague (*Yersinia pestis*)	A.D. 560	1894	1940s (antibiotics)
Polio (poliovirus)	A.D. 1885	1909 identified 1949 isolated	1953 (Salk vaccine)
AIDS (HIV)	A.D. 1981	1984	1986 (AZT partially effective)

Chapter 2). Table 11–1 shows a comparison of the time scales for fighting these diseases. Plague probably first caused major epidemics as early as the fifth or sixth century A.D.; the well-documented black deaths occurred in the fourteenth and following centuries A.D. The infectious agent, *Yersinia pestis*, was finally isolated in 1908. Effective therapy against the disease had to wait for the development of classical antibiotics in the 1940s.

Polio was first recognized as an epidemic disease in the 1880s, and the infectious agent, poliovirus, was isolated in the late 1940s. Even after the virus was identified, there was no effective therapy for individuals once they became infected. Ultimately, the disease was brought under control by the development of the Salk and Sabin polio vaccines beginning in 1955.

As for AIDS, the disease was first recognized in 1981 and the causative agent, HIV, was isolated in 1983–1984. By the end of 1986, the first partially effective antiviral, AZT, was developed; it was put into wide use in 1987. Thus, the rate of progress in AIDS research has actually been very rapid in historical terms.

The rapid progress in AIDS biomedical research largely reflects great advances in molecular biology, virology, immunology, and biotechnology that have taken place over the last 20 years. For instance, the life cycle of retroviruses was worked out largely in the 1970s, after the discovery of reverse transcriptase. In terms of immunology, the understanding of the different kinds of lymphocytes (B versus T; T_{killer} versus T_{helper}) is also quite recent. The techniques to identify the CD4 protein of T_{helper} lymphocytes are less than 15 years old. It is difficult to imagine how much more serious the AIDS epidemic would be if it had struck 20 years ago, before these advances. One program that provided a major boost to these fields was the war on cancer, which was a program launched by the U.S. federal government to conquer cancer with the same approach used to put a man on the moon. While the war on cancer has not been won yet, the program resulted in a great deal of research on retroviruses, and it heavily contributed to the development of recombinant DNA cloning technologies. This has been essential to the rapid achievements in AIDS research. The fact that biomedical research has advanced so rapidly in the last few years also makes us optimistic that new and more effective solutions to HIV and AIDS will be developed in the not-too-distant future.

In personal terms, there are positive approaches we all can take to dealing with the AIDS epidemic. Because death is an inevitable part of the lives of all of us, it is more productive to focus on wellness and the quality of life than on illness and death. This applies both to those who have AIDS and those who do not—as well as to people affected by cancer or other terminal illnesses. Like all major social changes, AIDS presents us not only with problems but also with opportunities on both biomedical and social levels. For example, we have already expanded our scientific knowledge of the immune system due to the efforts to understand AIDS. We also have a better understanding of the important factors in successful disease prevention and health promotion programs. There are many other opportunities to make progress on biological and social issues. AIDS is a crisis and an opportunity for social improvement: The challenge is to use the opportunities for greater personal, social, and biological understanding.

Glossary

ACT UP   Originally, the acronym for "AIDS Coalition to Unleash Power." Now, locally based, loosely organized associations of PWAs and their supporters.

AIDS   Acquired Immune Deficiency Syndrome is an incurable infectious viral disease that results in damage to the immune system in otherwise healthy individuals.

AIDS antibody test   A test to determine if an individual has antibodies to HIV, the virus that causes AIDS. Presence of HIV-specific antibodies indicates that the person has been exposed to HIV and has raised an immune response, but it does not tell if the person is still infected. The most common test is the ELISA test. A backup test called the Western blot is also used.

Analytical epidemiology   Epidemiological studies that seek to identify and explain the causes of diseases.

Anchoring   One judgment heuristic based on the starting point for an assessment and its effect on subsequent assessments.

Anonymous   A term used to describe HIV testing situations where the test results cannot be linked to an individual's name.

Antibiotics   Compounds that are effective against infection by microorganisms such as bacteria, fungi, and protozoa. They are generally ineffective against virus infections.

Antibody   A protein produced by a B-lymphocyte that specifically binds a particular antigen. This leads to attack by the immune system.

Antigen A molecule or substance against which a specific immune response is raised.

Antivirals Compounds that are effective in treating virus infections.

Asymptomatic AIDS carriers Individuals infected with HIV who do not show any sign of disease. They may be capable of infecting others.

Asymptomatic disease A disease for which there are no superficially visible or noticeable changes in the body or its functions which would indicate the presence of disease. (Contrast with **Symptomatic disease.**)

Attitude An individual's overall evaluation of information regarding people, objects, or issues.

Availability One judgment heuristic based on the presence of an item or object in memory. The two main components of availability are familiarity and salience.

Azidothymidine (AZT) Also called retrovir or zidovudine. An antiviral that is effective in treating HIV infection and AIDS. It works by preferentially inhibiting the action of reverse transcriptase during HIV replication.

Bacteria Small single-cell microorganisms that can cause diseases.

Behavior An individual's action regarding a specific issue.

B-lymphocytes One kind of lymphocyte. B-lymphocytes secrete antibodies that are specific for particular antigens.

Case/control studies A form of analtytical epidemiology in which a group of individuals with a particular disease (the cases) are compared to a matched group of unaffected individuals (the controls).

Case reports Reports and descriptions of an unusual disease occurrence in individual patients. Case reports are one form of descriptive epidemiology.

Causality The factors contributing to the development of disease in epidemiological studies.

CD4 protein   A surface protein that is characteristic of T_{helper} lymphocytes. It is also present on some macrophages. CD4 protein is the cell receptor for HIV.

Cellular immunity   Immunity involving T-lymphocytes (particularly T_{killer} lymphocytes).

Circulatory system   The system of vessels that moves blood around the body, including arteries, veins, and capillaries.

Cognition   A representation in an individual's mind arising from thinking or knowing.

Cognitive dissonance   An imbalance in cognitions caused by contradictions between elements of the cognitions. The imbalance creates psychological tension for resolution and the restoration of balance.

Cohort studies   A form of analytical epidemiology in which a group of individuals who share a particular risk factor for a disease are studied.

Confidential   A term used to describe HIV testing situations where the results are linked to an individual's name in an identifiable but protected way.

Control group   A group of individuals who serve as the scientific comparison for a similar but separate experimental group of individuals who receive a special treatment or intervention. The presence, meaning, and significance of changes in the experimental group due to the special treatment or intervention are identifiable through comparisons with the control group. See also **Experimental group**.

Cross-sectional/prevalence studies   Monitoring a population for occurrence of diseases and noting the time and kind of disease. A form of descriptive epidemiology.

Dementia   Loss of mental function due to damaged brain cells and brain inflammation in AIDS-afflicted patients.

Descriptive epidemiology   Epidemiological studies that describe the occurrence of disease by person, place, and time. Generally the first kinds of studies carried out in a new disease.

Discrimination   Behavior directed toward an individual based only on the individual's membership in a particular group.

ELISA   The most common test for HIV antibodies.

Endemic pattern   Patterns of continuous infection that allow epidemic diseases to remain present in populations.

Epidemiology   The study of patterns of disease occurrence in populations and the factors affecting them.

Experimental group   A group of individuals who receive a special treatment or intervention and who are compared with a control group of similar but separate individuals. See also **Control group**.

Experimental/interventional studies   A form of analytical epidemiology in which a condition in a population is changed, and the effect on disease development is observed.

Fotonovela (Spanish for "photo booklet")   A photo story book with pictures or sketches with captions in Spanish. Similar to a comic book in format.

Fungi   Microorganisms that may exist as single cells or be organized into simple multicellular organisms.

Germ theory   The postulate (1546) that infectious bacterial, fungal, or viral organisms cause disease.

Helper T-lymphocytes   T-lymphocytes that help T_{killer} and B-lymphocytes respond to antigens. Destruction of T_{helper} lymphocytes is the major problem in AIDS.

Heuristics   See **Judgment heuristics**.

HIV (Human Immunodeficiency Virus)   The virus that causes AIDS; previously called HTLV-III, LAV, and ARV. The predominant form of HIV in North America, Europe, and central Africa is called HIV-1. A closely related retrovirus found in western Africa is called HIV-2.

Hospice   An approach to caring for individuals in the terminal (or final) stages of an illness characterized by pain management instead of medical intervention and by attention to issues related to the individual in his/her social context (of family and friends).

Humoral immunity   Immunity involving B-lymphocytes and the antibodies they produce.

IDU   Injection drug user.

Immune system   The circulating cells and serum fluids in the blood that provide continuous protection from foreign infectious agents.

Immunological memory   The ability of the immune system to respond rapidly to a previously encountered antigen with specific antibodies.

Incidence   The proportion of a population that develops new cases of a disease during a particular time period.

Incubation period   The period between infection by a microorganism and appearance of disease symptoms.

Intention   An individual's decision to act in a particular manner regarding a specific issue. (Contrast this with **Behavior.**)

Judgment heuristics   Individualistic rules-of-thumb used in subjective probability models of decision making.

Kaposi's sarcoma   A normally rare cancer that develops frequently in AIDS patients.

Killer or cytotoxic T-lymphocytes   T-lymphocytes that kill the target cells they bind to.

Koch's postulates   A series of criteria used to establish that a particular microorganism causes a disease.

Latency   A state of virus infection in which the virus's genetic material remains hidden in the cell, but no virus is produced. At a later time, the latent virus may become reactivated. HIV can establish latent infection, particularly in macrophages.

Lentiviruses   A subclass of retroviruses that includes HIV. There are lentiviruses that infect other species, including monkeys, sheep, and cats.

Lymphadenopathy syndrome (LAS)   Persistently enlarged lymph nodes or swollen glands, sometimes an early sign of HIV infection that is progressing. Also called PGL (persistent generalized lymphadenopathy).

Lymphatic circulation   A second circulatory system that lymphocytes circulate through. Lymph channels drain fluid from tissues (lymph) into lymph nodes, where B- and T-lymphocytes are located. Antibodies or T-lymphocytes are produced in the lymph nodes in response to infection, and they enter the general circulation by way of other lymph channels.

Lymphocytes   Cells of the immune system that respond specifically to foreign substances. There are several kinds of lymphocytes. The two classes of lymphocytes are B-lymphocytes and T-lymphocytes.

Lymphoma   Cancer of lymphocytes of the immune system.

Lytic infection   Infection of a cell by a virus that results in death of the cell. HIV infection of T_{helper} lymphocytes is a lytic process.

Macrophages   One kind of phagocyte. Macrophages generally attack cells infected with viruses.

Non-lytic infection   Infection of a cell by a virus that results in production of virus, but survival of the cell. Most retroviruses normally carry out non-lytic infections. HIV infection of macrophages is non-lytic.

Norm   A standard about appropriate attitudes or behaviors for individuals or groups. The standard is socially defined or redefined, and it is maintained through social pressure. Some norms become formalized into laws, maintained through legal means.

Normative model   A decision-making approach that uses probabilistic information according to statistical rules to reach conclusions.

Opportunistic infections   Infections by common microorganisms that usually do not cause problems in healthy individuals. OIs are the major health problems for AIDS patients.

Optimistic bias   The tendency of an individual to believe that, compared to others, good things will happen to him and bad things will not happen.

Pandemic disease   An infectious disease present on many continents simultaneously.

Perceived severity   An individual's personal opinion about the severity of a disease. Perceived severity may or may not be closely related to actual severity (see **Severity**).

Perceived susceptibility   An individual's personal opinion about his/her susceptibility to a disease. Perceived susceptibility may or may not be closely related to actual susceptibility (see **Susceptibility**).

Personal invulnerability   The tendency of some individuals to believe that they are not susceptible to harmful risks. See **Optimistic bias.**

Phagocytes   Cells of the immune system that eat foreign cells or infected cells. There are two kinds of phagocytes: macrophages and neutrophils (granulocytes).

Prejudice   An unfavorable attitude toward a group of people.

Prevalence   The fraction of individuals in a population who have a disease or infection at a particular time.

Primary immune response   The immune response that follows exposure to an infection or an antigen for the first time. There is a lag period before antibodies are produced.

Probabilistic information   Material containing a statistical estimate related to an issue or topic.

Probability   A statistical estimate of likelihood, usually expressed as a proportion (from .00 to 1.00) or a percentage (from 0% to 100%).

Protozoa   Large single-cell microorganisms that can cause diseases.

PWA   Person with AIDS. **PWAs** are people with AIDS.

Red blood cells (erythrocytes)   Blood cells that are responsible for carrying oxygen and carbon dioxide to and from the tissues.

Representativeness   One judgment heuristic based on assumed similarity between two objects or items. One object or item is assumed to be representative of another to the extent that the two objects or items are similar.

Reverse transcriptase   An enzyme that is unique to all retroviruses. It reads the genetic information of the retrovirus, which is RNA, and makes a DNA copy.

Risk assessment   An evaluation of the susceptibility of a group or an individual to a particular threat (e.g., HIV infection).

Role   A position in a social setting involving interrelationships between and among people. An example would be the role of student, nurse, or patient.

Role expectations   The assumptions about the behaviors which an individual in a particular role will exhibit.

Schema   A combination of similar or related cognitions. Schemas serve as reference points for organizing an individual's past experiences or interpreting new experiences, or they serve as templates for activating new ideas.

Secondary immune response   An immune response that follows exposure to an infection or an antigen that the immune system has already encountered. The strength of the response is greater, it occurs more rapidly, and it lasts longer.

Self-concept   The schema an individual has about him- or herself. This self-schema is socially constructed and socially maintained.

Self-esteem   The positive or negative evaluation component of the self-concept.

Seronegative   An individual who tests negative for HIV antibodies.

Seropositive   An individual who tests positive for HIV antibodies.

Severity   Seriousness of a disease in terms of causing unpleasant or harmful effects on the body, possibly to the point of being life-threatening. (See also **Perceived severity**.)

Stereotype   Group-based schema generally reflecting society's appraisal of the group. Stereotypes can be either positive or negative.

Stigma   A negative assessment associated with a particular object or issue.

Subjective probability model   A decision-making approach that uses probabilistic information according to individualistic, personal biases to reach conclusions.

Surrogate endpoint   Indicators of the effectiveness of drug therapies which substitute for the standard indicators (i.e., development of disease or death). For HIV, surrogate endpoints are measures of the condition of an individual's immune system such as CD4 lymphocyte counts and the amount of viral protein (p24 antigen) in the blood.

Susceptibility   Capacity of a person to be infected by or to be unresistant to a disease. (Contrast with **Perceived susceptibility**.)

Symptomatic disease   A disease for which there are superficially visible or noticeable changes in the body or its functions which indicate the presence of the disease. These changes are unpleasant or harmful and thus call attention to the consequences of the disease. (Contrast with **Asymptomatic disease**.)

Test group   See **Experimental group**.

T-lymphocytes   One kind of lymphocyte. Unlike B-lymphocytes, T-lymphocytes do not release antibodies, but they specifically recognize and bind foreign antigens. There are two main types of T-lymphocytes: T_{killer} and T_{helper} lymphocytes.

Vaccine   A killed or harmless microorganism that can induce an immune response to a disease-causing agent. This will confer protection against the disease-causing agent in uninfected people. This is the major preventative measure against viral infections.

Viral envelopes   Structures that surround some virus particles, resembling membranes around cells. Viral envelopes contain virus-specific proteins that are important in binding cell receptors. Viral envelope proteins are major targets for the immune system.

Viruses   Small infectious agents. They are parasites that must grow inside cells.

Western blot   An HIV antibody test, used as a confirmatory test for a positive ELISA test.

White blood cells (leukocytes)   All blood cells except red blood cells. Leukocytes consist of a variety of blood cells including lymphocytes, neutrophils, eosinophils, macrophages, and mega-karyocytes.

Window period   For an individual, the period of time between infection by a virus and the production of antibodies to the virus.

Xenophobia   Discriminatory fear of foreigners.

Index